Healing
NIGHT

~

the SCIENCE *and* SPIRIT
of *Sleeping, Dreaming,* and *Awakening*

Healing
NIGHT

~

the SCIENCE *and* SPIRIT
of *Sleeping, Dreaming,* and *Awakening*

RUBIN R. NAIMAN, Ph.D.

SYREN BOOK COMPANY
MINNEAPOLIS

Published by
Syren Book Company
5120 Cedar Lake Road
Minneapolis, MN 55416

Printed in the United States of America on acid-free paper

ISBN-13: 978-0-929636-53-5
ISBN-10: 0-929636-53-8

LCCN 2005933853

Cover design by Kyle G. Hunter
Book design by Ann Sudmeier

To my mother and father ⌒
MOLLIE AND CHARLES NAIMAN

You, darkness, of whom I am born—

I love you more than the flame
that limits the world
to the circle it illumines
and excludes all the rest.

But the dark embraces everything:
shapes and shadows, creatures and me,
people, nations—just as they are.

It lets me imagine
a great presence stirring beside me.

I believe in the night.

—RAINER MARIA RILKE

Contents

Foreword

Hugh Prather

THROUGHOUT MANY YEARS OF COUNSELING OTHERS, I have been struck by how consistently we humans discount our darkness. In contrast, Dr. Rubin Naiman fully acknowledges the importance of darkness and loves the sacredness of night. He sees with uncanny clarity the function that falling asleep, deep sleep, dreaming, and awakening play in our relationships, our careers, the daily grind, and, above all, our spiritual growth.

My own appreciation of sleep began many years ago when I tried maintaining conscious awareness throughout the hypnagogic state, that period of mind-altering drowsiness preceding sleep. I eventually noted that there is a natural and rejuvenating relinquishment of the ego as we descend into deep sleep.

A few years later, I tried to more carefully observe the hypnopompic state—that half-conscious state that precedes complete awakening. These observations confirmed that the sleep-relinquished ego is then downloaded anew each morning. We are presented with a choice at this time either to continue operating on automatic pilot or to break with our past and plug into our deeper core. If we open to it, we are faced with the important question of what identity we will assume when we awaken.

Rubin Naiman and I have had many lunchtime discussions about phenomena such as these, and always I have come away from these conversations realizing that I have received more insight than I have given. His capacity to empathize and connect within his own personal life adds a new dimension to his inspired theories. In contrast to traditional approaches to sleep, Naiman's work is based not only on clinical experience and scientific research but also on his personal explorations. As you wade into the mystical pool of sleep investigation, you will sense that this subject has been Naiman's passion for decades. This book is unquestionably a labor of love, and like love, it expands the mind as well as the heart.

Unlike the authors of most of the books and papers I have read about dreaming, Naiman does not traditionally analyze dream symbols. Rather, he uses the reader's personal narrative as a tool to unlock the mysteries of dreams and dreaming. Instead of asking what does the dream tell us about our life, he poses this startling question: "If our life were already a dream, what does dreaming tell us about who we are?"

Perhaps the greatest benefit this book bestows is a fuller understanding of the sacredness of the dark side of day and the importance of the shadow side of human nature. Naiman brilliantly uses circadian rhythms—the play of darkness and light—as symbol and even synonym for our higher and lower selves. *Healing Night* is a book of enlightenment that not only inspires and informs but also provides effective means for our own transformations. The reader feels respected and cared for within the covers of this book. I give you this promise. After reading this book, you will not be the same person you were.

Preface

IN RECENT DECADES, sleep disorders have emerged as the most prevalent health concern in the industrialized world, affecting not only our health, welfare, and safety but also our very consciousness. Although important strides are being made in understanding sleep from a scientific and medical standpoint, we have failed to acknowledge the broader environmental and psychospiritual context of our sleep. We have failed to acknowledge night.

Our approach to sleep medicine, which is born of modern culture, is severely constrained by its mechanical presumptions. We see ourselves as machines. Consequently, the solutions we seek for our damaged sleep are naïve and overly mechanistic, primarily involving chemical switching mechanisms. Getting to sleep is about switching off, and waking up is about switching back on. As a result, we have come to depend excessively on sleep medications, alcohol, and substances to buffer our encounter with night—and on caffeine, sugar, adrenaline, and "waking pills" to maintain a steady charge throughout the day.

Healing Night is about restoring a sense of sacredness to our nights and night consciousness. To do so, we must reconsider our contemporary, limited conception of sleep, which has been stripped of its natural and spiritual context. When we speak of sleep, we must recognize that we cannot reasonably segregate it from dreaming and awakening. The rhythmic flow of sleep, dreams, and awakening must, furthermore, be considered in its natural context of night—of dusk, darkness, and dawn. Only such an inclusive perspective of night consciousness will allow us to transcend the constraints of our overly mechanistic view and open the way to a more meaningful, effective, and personally enriching approach to night.

The official emblem of the American Academy of Sleep Medicine, the foremost professional sleep organization in the United States, is a modified Taoist yin-yang symbol. It serves as an apt representation of the central role of rhythms—of the pulse of night and day, of darkness and light—in understanding sleep. Reminding us also of the essential unity behind duality, above all, the yin-yang serves as a universal symbol of spirituality. Ironically, sleep medicine makes absolutely no allowance for the spiritual dimensions of night, sleep, or dreams.

Night is home to a delicate spirituality. Its sleep and dreams cannot be reduced to squiggly EEG tracings and the complex cascade of bodily humors. As we will see, there is a lovely, sacred, and mythic dimension to our night consciousness. Our challenge is to appreciate the mechanisms of sleep, dreams, and awakening without sacrificing their essential spiritual qualities. Reconsidering night in this way calls upon us to reevaluate and redefine what we deem "normal" in sleep, dreams, and waking.

Healing Night offers a new way of looking at sleeping, dreaming, and awakening that tempers scientific knowledge with spiritual sensitivity. Although the book draws heavily on empirical knowledge and clinical experience, it does not sacrifice what is deeply subjective and mystical. In contrast to the sterile, overly clinical approach of contemporary sleep medicine, *Healing Night* provides a much-needed alternative that is both integrative and personal. It is written for anyone interested in night consciousness, including people concerned with sleep problems. Toward this end, most chapters finish with suggestions for practices to help heal sleep disturbances.

But *Healing Night* does not offer yet another shortsighted, quick mechanical fix. Simplistic laundry lists of suggestions for improving one's sleep abound. At best, these offer stopgap measures. At worst, they can damage our sleep and dreams by misleading us into relating to night in the same way we manage day, distracting us from the deeper, nonordinary world of night consciousness.

By reconsidering sleeping, dreaming, and awakening in their natural home of night, *Healing Night* explores darkness itself as a potent sleep medicine. And it encourages us to reexamine and heal our deeply denied yet very palpable fear of the dark.

Healing Night, as we shall see, is also about healing our days. If we allow ourselves an honest and sober encounter with darkness, we will begin to see sleeping, dreaming, and waking in a whole new way. In fact, we could begin to see in whole a new way.

September 2005
Tucson, Arizona

Acknowledgments

I HAVE BEEN BLESSED with many guides and teachers who have nurtured my personal and professional growth. I extend my heartfelt gratitude to Stephen Levine; Hugh Prather; Chuck Rastatter, Ed.D.; Tom Steiner, Ph.D.; Jesse Stoff, M.D.; and James Stewart; and to the spirit of Elisabeth Kübler-Ross, M.D.

Andrew Weil, M.D., Victoria Maizes, M.D., Randy Horrowitz, M.D., Ph.D., and the faculty and fellows at the University of Arizona's Program in Integrative Medicine have provided a safe, stimulating, and especially nourishing professional home for my work in integrative sleep medicine. I am deeply grateful to all of them.

My patients have also been my teachers. I am thankful for their lessons in courage, faith, and healing. I am also indebted to the staff and guests at Canyon Ranch Health Resort and Miraval Resort in Tucson for invaluable teaching and learning opportunities around my work in sleep and dreams.

For their meaningful and timely encouragement, I offer my deep appreciation to Thomas Cahill; Betty Sue Flowers, Ph.D.; Melanie Grimes, RSHom (NA), CCH; Nancy Hand; Kathleen Johnson, R.D.; Maya Levanon; Susan Pack; Russell Pierce, Ph.D.; Carolyn Ross, M.D.; Anthony Skinner, Ph.D.; and Janice Warne.

Many, many thanks to those who nurtured and edited my work. Amy Weintraub expertly and gently ushered me into the world of writing. Susan Raihoffer and Maria Manske provided essential organizational guidance for this book. And Teryn Johnson, Robin Fasano, and Mary Keirstead shared the challenging task of expertly editing my work. Behind the scenes, Stefanie Marlis, Arthur Naiman, Marla Paul, Karen Thomas, and Lori Weiss all provided insight and support.

For their commitment and kindness, I extend my love and deep appreciation to Tim Collins, Marc Gold, David Hochner, Harry Kressler, Terry Real, Rocky Smolin, Marsha Sutton, Heide Weisel, and Jack Weisel. My sons, Jesse, Daniel, and Zachary Naiman, have contributed much more than they will ever know to this book, as has my lovely granddaughter, Claire. I am most grateful for her lessons in innocence and inspiration. Special thanks to Sam and Evelyn Nerenblatt and to Merrill "Bubby" Eisenberg. Hugh and Gayle Prather offered loving and expert guidance and support in more ways than I can recount. I am most grateful for their presence in my life.

Finally, I am appreciative to all the weird and wondrous life forms at the Epic Café, Bentley's, and the B-Line for providing me with a real world place to think, write, talk, and eat—and for their incomparable decaffeinated concoctions.

Introduction

"WHAT IS THE BEST THING IN THE WORLD?" asked my mother.

When I was a young boy, she played a curious game with me. Somehow it did not matter that we had played it out countless times before, that I already knew the right answer, and that I would once again tease her with childish responses I knew she would dismiss. The fact that she was smiling and in a playful mood was reason enough for me to engage her.

My first answer was always, "Ice cream!"

"No," she smiled.

"Then cartoons!" I said.

"No."

"Toys!"

"No, no." She laughed and shook her head.

"What then?" I shouted through my giggles.

"Night," said my mother. "Night is the best thing in the world!"

I would continue to argue through laughter and large gestures, trying to explain how daytime was so much better because you mostly slept at night. But she held firm.

As the years passed and I was able to better understand my mother's traumatic history as a teenager in a Nazi concentration camp, I came to know that she meant it. Night was the best thing in the world. She *loved* the night. And, just as much, she loved sleep—dreams and all. Somehow, theories of posttraumatic stress disorder notwithstanding, she managed to sleep and dream well—very well, in fact.

Throughout her years of struggle as a prisoner of war, the descent of dusk routinely brought a most welcomed truce. Receding light softened and quieted the outer world of toil and suffering. And, as the bustle of day slowed and eventually stopped, there came an opportunity for a sweet surrender into the safe arms of darkness.

Night brought sleep—a vital daily measure of peace. Sleep, in turn, served as a natural bridge to dreams. And dreaming opened a mysterious portal to a more malleable and compassionate reality. Dreams offered a simple reminder of something cruelly unavailable by day—a sense of possibility, a sense of hope.

Night Blindness

We suffer today from serious complications of *psychospiritual night blindness*—a far-reaching failure to understand the significance of night in our lives, health, and spirituality. Over the past century, "civilized" nights have grown significantly shorter. A culture of zealous industrialization has polluted the night environment with excessive and pernicious artificial illumination. Blinded by this light, we have lost our regard for the natural milieu of dusk, dawn, and the intervening darkness of night. Daylight has been deified and darkness demonized. It would seem that even as adults, *we are afraid of the dark.*

And we are losing sleep over it. Inundated by day, we suffer by night from an unprecedented epidemic of sleep disorders that take a substantial toll on our health, well-being, and productivity. Our negation of night is further complicated by widespread damage to our dream lives—a literal and figurative loss of our dreams. Like sleep loss, dream loss affects virtually all aspects of our lives, especially our personal sense of spirituality. A less obvious but equally serious casualty of our night blindness is a common proclivity for weary and mindless morning awakenings that have subtle but disturbing repercussions on the quality of our daily lives.

Disordered sleep, suppressed dreams, and disturbed awakenings all tangle together into a dense obstruction of awareness. By day, we experience ourselves and the world around us through a depleted and dulled sensorium. Our very consciousness is damaged and downsized. We lose sight of the bigger picture, our peripheral vision, our imagination. Far too many of us live in a kind of foggy bubble—a chronic, low-grade, and insidious daze. But, somehow, we manage to conjure sufficient energy to maintain our relentless drive.

The global energy crisis seems to have a curious internal representation—a personal energy crisis. Our chronic depletion results in an insatiable hunger for personal energy. To compensate for our sleep- and dream-deprived daze and maintain our frenetic drive, we reflexively spike our waking hours with *counterfeit energies*. We are a society of energy addicts, with lifestyles designed to provide us with quick fixes of caffeine and sugar on demand. Or, more subtly, as we will see, with overstimulating information and excessive light at night. Unfortunately, such energy spikes inevitably backfire with jittery withdrawals. Our desperate need for rest, then, is met only with a sputtering restlessness that conceals an underlying exhaustion. Beyond damaging our waking consciousness, the use of counterfeit energies further damages our nights by disrupting nature's essential rhythm of activity and rest.

But we can take something for it. Evening appears to be the most common period of substance and medication use in our world. We consume vast amounts of alcohol, marijuana, antidepressants, sleeping pills, and tranquilizers to modulate our restless waking energies, and, even more so, to blunt our uneasy encounter with dusk and darkness. These substances may help us temporarily negotiate our discomfort with night, but only at a terrible cost. Many of us routinely view the night only through bleary eyes.

Unfortunately, what is called *sleep medicine*—that branch of the health sciences specialized to treat sleep disorders—offers little help with our night blindness. By tightly framing night, sleep, and dreams as strictly objective and scientific phenomena, sleep specialists drain these experiences of anything personal or subjective, let alone sacred or spiritual. Sadly, sleep medicine also segregates sleep from her biological sib, dreaming, consigning the latter to the status of unappreciated stepchild. (It is, after all, *sleep* medicine, not *sleep and dream* medicine.) Most sleep specialists relegate what is left of night to autonomic mechanisms—reducing sleeping and dreaming to molecular machinations that are about as personally meaningful as recharging a battery.

Viewed through such a narrow and rigid lens, sleep and dreams become experiences we believe we can and must manipulate and control. We seek medical and mechanical solutions to what are essentially lifestyle and consciousness problems. In lieu of an honest confrontation with our frenetic drive and fear of darkness, we are offered a tantalizing array of designer sleeping and waking pills. In bed with the pharmaceutical industry, sleep medicine itself remains in a fitful, dream-deprived sleep.

More than three decades ago Andrew Weil called our attention to the concept of nighttime consciousness. In his book *The Marriage of the Sun and Moon,* he explored the innate, universal human drive to experience nonordinary forms of consciousness. To balance our ordinary waking, daytime, or "solar consciousness," Dr. Weil encouraged us to intentionally open to a darker, more mysterious night, or "lunar consciousness." Lunar, or night consciousness encompasses sleep and dreams but also includes dark or shadowy aspects of waking awareness.

As a culture, we have failed to achieve the necessary balance between these separate but equally important realms of consciousness. "Like night and day," solar and lunar consciousnesses have become increasingly polarized. Daylight is dominant, overvalued, and even deified, while darkness is dismissed, devalued, and often demonized. From divine light to light beer, things associated with the metaphor of light suggest goodness. We want to shed light, see the light, and lighten up. Our associations with metaphoric darkness, on the other hand, are suggestive of confusion, struggle, immorality, and outright evil. We want nothing more than to avoid dark times, dark nights of the soul, and, of course, the dreaded "prince of darkness."

Our struggle with night is ultimately a struggle with denied aspects of our own darkness. Confusing the literal darkness of night with the metaphoric darkness of life, we blindly project our feelings about the latter onto the former. We then mitigate our fear of darkness through the excessive use of evening light, effectively extending daytime's custody over us deep into the night and seriously eroding our night consciousness. Indoors and out, our nights are lit up beyond reason—so far beyond what necessity and safety might dictate. Like a frightened child, the planet sleeps with its lights on.

In the end, sleep and dream disorders are largely symptomatic of this deeper fear of night and its damaging segregation from day. In our attempt to excise darkness from our lives, our very consciousness has been cleaved. With the loss of night, day loses its partner in the sacred dance of circadian cycles. Adam loses Eve. Yin is torn from yang. And activity becomes dangerously devoid of rest. We lose our sense of the basic pulse of night and day—our precious awareness of life's natural rhythms. Ultimately, we lose our experience of the lovely, seamless continuity of consciousness, our sense of oneness.

An Integrative Approach

Healing Night is different in scope from most contemporary takes on sleep, dreams, and their related problems. It is meant to lay a foundation for a new approach, one that is, in the broadest sense of the term, *integrative*. Although it wholeheartedly supports the integration of conventional medical approaches with those of complementary and alternative medicine, this work is primarily concerned with an even more fundamental integration, that of the segregated aspects of our consciousness. Truly effective strategies for preventing and healing sleep and dream disorders are hampered by the absence of such an approach.

An integrative approach seeks to reaffirm the marriage of the sun and moon. This sacred union restores the essential connectedness and continuity of sleeping, dreaming, and awakening. We cannot meaningfully understand these experiences independently of one another and outside of the larger context of their daily rhythmic sweep through our lives. In recognizing their continuity, an integrative approach reinstates a critical sense of something desperately lacking in our highly mechanized and driven world: nature's fundamental rhythmicity.

An integrative approach invites subjectivity back into science. It recognizes the importance of personal and social meaning as a balance to hard science's overly objective posture toward night consciousness. In doing so, it acknowledges, considers, and respects the legitimacy of the personal experiences of sleeping, dreaming, and awakening. Essentially, it restores consciousness itself to night.

An integrative approach also incorporates spirit back into science. It calls for complementing sleep medicine's objectivity with a depth psychological and traditional, sacred view of night consciousness. Such a spiritual perspective of night is certainly not new. Regard for sacred dimensions of night and night consciousness is found in all major Eastern and Western religious traditions, including Hinduism, Buddhism, Judaism, Christianity, and Islam. Ancient and indigenous spiritual beliefs and practices, as well as metaphysical teachings, also acknowledge the sanctity of darkness, sleeping, dreaming, and awakening. For example, Rudolf Steiner, the prolific nineteenth-century Austrian philosopher, lectured extensively and passionately about the critical role of sleep and dreams in spiritual life.

The integration of sleep science with personal meaning and spiritual perspectives opens the way to a more expansive, magnificent, and mythic vision of night, a vision that will both clarify the central challenge of our fear of darkness and simultaneously map our journey toward its healing.

Nightmindedness

Nyx, the forgotten primordial Greek goddess of night, is calling for resurrection. And there are unexpected gifts to be found in the darkness she brings, if we choose to be more *nightminded*. Night has been celebrated and sanctified with rich social and sacred rituals across cultures and time. Whether it is the initial transition through dusk, the experience of sleeping and dreaming, or the coming of dawn and awakening, each phase of night offers sacred and healing possibilities. And, as we will see, a more honest relationship with night also offers vital lessons about our need to rest by day.

Perhaps the greatest gift of becoming more nightminded is the restoration of a kind of night vision—a fundamentally different way of seeing or perceiving. Because sleeping, dreaming, and awakening are nonordinary states of consciousness, their exploration calls for nonordinary ways of perceiving—a kind of *nocturnal lucidity*. Nocturnal lucidity is a way of seeing in the dark, a kind of third-eye sightedness. We can clearly see night only through such a spiritual wide-angle lens. And when applied to our view of day, this expanded frame restores a sense of the big picture to our lives. It restores the numinous.

Having survived the Holocaust, my mother learned to distinguish the literal darkness of night from metaphoric darkness— what has been referred to as *shadow*. Certainly one does not have to suffer from posttraumatic stress disorder, or anguish in any form, to receive the gifts of night. They are available to all.

Night itself is the best sleep medicine. We cannot heal our sleep and dream disorders without first healing our relationship with night. And in healing night, we discover that night itself is healing. Darkness is a healing retreat, a carbon filter for the soul. It is safe to sigh at night. If we surrender to it, the night will inhale our shadowy fears, offering precious personal insights in return. Beyond all of the psychological and biomedical complexities associated with it, we come to discover that sleep itself is a spiritual path, dreaming a means of walking this path, and awakening its gracious gift. We come to learn that there is something we can safely place our faith in—even in the dark.

⌒

Healing Night is divided into ten chapters. Chapters 1 and 2 provide an overview of the problems associated with the loss of night as well as a basic framework for understanding night consciousness. The core of the book, chapters 3, 4, 5, and 6, provide a detailed excursion into the problems and potentials of sleeping, dreaming, and awakening. The waking expressions of night consciousness, including a discussion of waking, shadow, and the waking dream, are considered in chapters 7, 8, and 9. And finally, chapter 10 offers recommendations for our collective healing of night as well as a new conceptual framework for an integrative understanding of sleeping, dreaming, and waking.

～1

Let There Be Night

Not the city light. We want
—the moon—
The Moon
none of our own doing!

—RAE ARMANTROUT

ALMOST EVERYWHERE ON OUR PLANET, night bears little resemblance to how it looked just one century ago. Although the electric light bulb was invented in the late 1800s, it was used quite sparingly for decades after. Even as late as 1950, 70 percent of rural households in the United States still had no electric lighting.

In times past, human activity naturally downshifted as dusk signaled the approach of night. There was no rush to get home since most people were already there. A majority of Americans were still living and working in rural areas. As daylight gradually receded, the winds would quiet, and the rhythmic chirp of crickets and night birds began as all things darkened, cooled, and slowed.

Evening activities occurred in a much gentler, dimmer light and were usually relaxing and restful. Dinnertime depended less on the clock and more on the season, on nature's timing. Rather than watching television, catching up on work, drinking, and being entertained, people made a slow and easy transition toward sleep.

Reinforcing this lifestyle were various religious and folk traditions that rendered night, sleeping, and dreaming more personally meaningful. Evening contemplative practices prepared one for bed, sleep, and dreams. Storytelling, day's end prayers, and the study of sacred texts would slow one's pace and gently invite an inward focus. The Bible, which is centered on a simpler time, was commonly read in the evenings. Here sleep and dreams are treated with interest and deep regard. In fact, the second creation story in Genesis begins with Adam falling asleep.

Recent historical studies of how people slept in preindustrial times as well as related scientific findings have raised interesting questions about what might actually constitute a truly natural human sleep pattern. Bedtime occurred not too long after dark and was approached with considerably more receptivity than we bring to it today. It appears that people struggled less with falling asleep, even if sleep did not arrive on cue. Evidence suggests that in earlier centuries extended middle-of-the-night awakenings were not necessarily looked upon as disordered sleep. In fact, as we will see, such awakenings appear to have been common and regarded as normal, natural occurrences that held important personal, social, and even spiritual value.

First morning light and the crowing of a cock gently signaled a natural rising time. Morning routines depended less on the hour and minute and more on the natural, biological needs of people and their domestic animals. The day was not structured by clock and culture but by rhythm and nature. In America today, except for the rare unregulated camping trip—usually too short to matter—individuals can live a lifetime without ever experiencing a body and soul that is truly in sync with nature's rhythms.

As dusk approaches, typical modern nights begin with *rush hour*—a massive, noisy, grinding, and smoky movement of people and machines. Automobiles, motorcycles, buses, trains, and planes shuttle millions of people from places of work, school, and daily errands back to their homes. In actuality, rush hour does not live up to its name. The rush is only in intention since traffic is hopelessly congested in most major metropolitan areas. Nor does it last an hour. Recent studies indicate the average length of evening traffic congestion in these metropolitan areas is actually closer to three hours.

Rush hour may be as much a personal psychological challenge

as it is a public transport predicament. With a formal end to the day's activities, we commonly experience the emotional gridlock of unfinished business, unmet needs, and unprocessed feelings held back throughout the busy day. Often, we simply cannot afford to slow or stop just because the sun has decided to set.

We generally fail to notice the onset of night. As daylight recedes, lights immediately come on everywhere—commercial lights, office lights, streetlights, headlights. We are clearly in mass denial that something hemispheric and profound is occurring. For millions who want to slow but have trouble with the inertia of high-speed days, chemical emergency brakes are readily available in the form of alcohol, tranquilizers, and drugs. Rush hour is conveniently complemented by "happy hour." In bars, clubs, or our homes we can immerse ourselves in myriad distractions to complement our substance-induced daze. And if coming to a full stop for dinner is not possible, we have the option of fast food to match our pace.

As we reach our homes, more lights come on. Porch lights, house lights, and television sets. For those who elect not to be taken out by a happy-hour haze, evenings can be bustling: time to catch up, time for family, friends, neglected kids, unfinished projects, voice mail, e-mail, unpaid bills, lapsed exercise programs, and an amazing array of entertainment options. While everything around us in the natural world is yielding to darkness, many of us are anticipating a second wind.

In recent decades the naturally quieting influence of dusk has been displaced by the cultural imperative of "prime time," most certainly a key factor in epidemic sleep and dream disturbances. Prime time literally primes us—but not for sleep. To comply with expectations that we remain fully alert if not completely active into the evening, we boost our naturally slumping energies with foods, substances, and activities. We refuel with caffeine, refined sugars, adrenaline, and, yes, gratuitous evening light. Rather than allowing ourselves to gradually let go of the day, we extend an active, waking, daytime posture into the start of night. In fact, we extend daylight itself.

If God, angels, or extraterrestrials were indeed monitoring us from above, the most profound change they would have witnessed on this planet since its creation is the metastatic illumination of our nights. We have responded to the quieting offer of night with an innervating program of excessive artificial illumination. This includes an astounding average of four hours of nightly television. Our celestial observers might find it curious that with the arrival of night we continue to gaze intently, almost longingly, upon electronically reconstituted images of a daytime world, all lit up, fully animated, and wide awake.

Our nights have grown significantly shorter. When God said, "Let there be light," He divided it equally with night. But when Edison said, "Let there be even more light," he appropriated it from night. And there are serious casualties in what has escalated into an undeclared war against dusk and darkness. Despite the fact that shift work is known to present serious health and mental health risks, no fewer than 25 million American workers have been assigned to patrol the occupied territory. In addition to its deleterious effects on sleep, overexposure to nighttime illumination has also been linked to increases in cancer, diabetes, and immune dysfunctions—giving new meaning to the notion of friendly fire.

So much of our use of light at night is gratuitous. The light bulb, originally designed to extend the workday, has ignited the landscape and is now burning out of control. Widespread blazes visible from outer space continue to engulf growing portions of the planet's surface, emitting another kind of pollutant that presents an insidious danger. Because it interferes with the ability to study celestial bodies, astronomers were the first to raise concerns about night-sky light pollution. The International Dark Sky Association, an interdisciplinary professional organization concerned with global light pollution, has compiled compelling evidence suggesting that light at night (LAN) is overused, an unnecessary energy and economic burden, and detrimental to the environment and health. Beyond wasting immense amounts of electrical power, light pollution is damaging plant life, killing birds, and, as we will see, compromising human health.

Light, of course, is a primary form of energy and will variously

energize or excite whatever it makes contact with—including humans. Excessive LAN promises excessive artificial stimulation, a
major source of the counterfeit energy that fuels so much of our
evening wakefulness. Mounting evidence suggests that even moderate nighttime light exposure can delay and suppress our biological drive to sleep in a matter of days. What might it do over
decades? I believe that habitual use of excessive LAN is the most
important overlooked factor in our contemporary sleep and dream
disorders epidemic.

Like our celestial observers, as passengers flying over the civilized landscape at night, we see below us numerous eerily illuminated enclaves of hyperactivity on the part of one species only.
Everywhere else life, in rhythm with the rotation of the earth, is
slowing, cooling, and quieting.

Disordered Sleep

Somehow, we do manage to quiet and slow. And we make it to
sleep. Or do we? Sleep disorders are the most prevalent health
concern in America and probably the rest of the industrialized
world today. Through ongoing rigorous surveys of sleep patterns
in the United States, the National Sleep Foundation (1994–2005)
has gathered revealing data on Americans' habits and struggles
around sleep. Their findings suggest that a majority of American
adults experience regular symptoms of sleep disorders. These include chronic patterns of insufficient sleep, various forms of insomnia, sleep-related breathing disorders, as well as a host of other
serious problems that compromise sleep quantity and quality. Sleep
scientists have identified nearly one hundred specific sleep disorders that afflict our nights.

The National Sleep Foundation (2005) found that 75 percent
of American adults experienced symptoms of sleep problems at
least a few nights per week. Many millions of us routinely struggle
with insomnia—difficulties with falling asleep, staying asleep, or
maintaining quality sleep throughout the night. The incidence of
insomnia is, furthermore, steadily rising.

Sixty million Americans chronically struggle with insufficient sleep syndrome, an overriding compulsion to trade sleep for productivity. During the past three decades alone, Americans have increased their net work time by an average of one full month per year, the equivalent of about 150 extra hours of work. The situation is even worse for working mothers, who in the same period of time have increased their work time by about six weeks a year.

With the growth in popularity of electric lighting, Americans lost nearly 20 percent of their sleep time—nearly a two-hour cut per night. Compared to the turn of the past century, when they were obtaining about nine hours nightly, Americans today are sleeping an average of about seven hours per night. In fact, about 30 percent of adults obtain six hours or less of sleep per night. The average sleep time of adolescents and college students has also plummeted in recent years, decreasing about two hours per night.

There is strong, mounting evidence that lost and damaged sleep is associated with a wide range of serious medical and psychiatric conditions. A number of studies have linked the loss of deep sleep to the contemporary epidemic of obesity. Additional research suggests that those who obtain an average of only six hours of sleep per night increase their risk of viral infection by 50 percent. Still other studies suggest that habitual short sleepers, people who sleep less than five or six hours per night, have significantly higher rates of coronary heart disease. An American Cancer Society study including one million participants confirmed that short sleepers had not only higher incidences of fatal heart disease and stroke but also significantly higher incidences of cancers across the board. We will take a closer look at an interesting theoretical connection between dreaming and cancer as we proceed.

The link between sleep and mental health is critical and complex. Approximately 80 percent of people with mental health problems also suffer from insomnia. Although sleep disorders are a common symptom of mental health problems, they also appear to be causal factors. Insomnia, for example, has long been known to be a classic symptom of depression. In recent years sleep scientists have confirmed that insomnia is also a major cause of depression.

Sleeping and dreaming affect our psychological well-being, influencing our moods, attention, learning, and memory.

To complicate matters further, what we commonly consider normal sleep may not be. Our mechanistic view of sleep leads us to confuse being asleep with being unconscious. Too often we believe we are obtaining deep and restorative sleep when, in fact, we are simply knocked out by medications, substances, or the backlash of sleep deprivation. As we shall see, such mistaken beliefs perpetuate our night blindness and further exacerbate our sleep disorders.

Disordered Dreaming

We are at least as dream deprived as we are sleep deprived. Given the common tendency to lump sleep and dreams together, many of the symptoms attributed to sleep loss may actually result from suppressed dreaming.

Dreams, dreaming, and their daytime analogue, the *waking dream,* are devalued in modern life. We too casually accept the fact that many widely used substances and medications significantly suppress dreaming. The dream is, furthermore, being gradually displaced by the dramatic, where all sorts of entertaining distractions are substituted for dreaming. With the chronic suppression of dreams, the color is slowly bleached from our lives, contributing to depression—waking life devoid of its naturally expansive dreamy context. And, as we will see, with the loss of our night dreams, we lose touch with our waking dreams, with the larger world of the creative, sacred, and imaginal process.

In contrast to rich folk, spiritual, and psychological traditions that ascribe value and meaning to dreams and dreaming, contemporary science has diverted our attention almost exclusively to the physiological and functional aspects of dreaming. Despite the fact that dreaming is as different from sleeping as is waking, sleep science minimizes dreaming by subsuming it under sleep. Dreaming is seen merely as another stage of sleep. It is "paradoxical *sleep*" or "REM *sleep*." And dreams are reduced to a biology of REM, the rapid eye movements that usually accompany them by night.

Through the frozen eyes of neuroscience, the process of dreaming is strictly functional, and dreams themselves are viewed as nothing more than bits of neurological flotsam and jetsam—meaningless by-products of the brain's nightly housecleaning.

Too many children learn early that dreams, as well as their waking expression through imagination, are of limited value in the "real" world. They are simply not real. As adults, our consensual reality dictates that we define our "dreams" as something we pursue through work—not dream work. We live lives that are ever more hopelessly entrenched in the mundane.

The defensive posture toward dreaming reflected in Hamlet's classic "to sleep per chance to dream" may be more relevant today than ever. Millions of people appear to awaken at night in reaction to the onset of dreaming. Some of what we call *sleep maintenance insomnia* might more accurately be thought of as *dream onset insomnia*. Many of us know intuitively that what we deny and repress by day will emerge opportunistically by night, often through our dreams. And we would rather it not.

Our bodies and minds need to dream and will find ways of doing so. Scientific experiments that selectively inhibit animals or humans from dreaming routinely result in a pressured *dream rebound*. This rebound is also experienced by the millions of people whose dreaming is suppressed by alcohol, drugs, and many common prescription medications. After a period of suppressed dreaming, we are likely to dream more, more intensely, and earlier in our sleep cycles. Suppressed dreams can rebound with a vengeance, resulting in nightmares and insomnia. Highly pressured dream rebounds can also displace deep sleep and, as we will see later, even intrude into waking consciousness.

Increased pressure to dream is also strongly correlated with depression. Numerous studies confirm that depressed people frequently experience increased dreaming as well as the premature appearance of dreams in their nightly sleep cycles. Interestingly, virtually all antidepressant medications will, to varying degrees, suppress dreaming. It is astounding that modern psychiatry has actually come to view dreaming as a symptom that needs to be suppressed in the treatment of depression. From a more traditional psychodynamic perspective, depression has long been understood in terms of a symbolic loss of one's dreams. Is it not more feasible that dreaming is a natural process through which the mind attempts to heal itself?

Entertainment, the new opiate of the masses, mitigates the subtle ache and numbness symptomatic of our dream loss. Our innate hunger for the imaginative and creative sustenance of dreaming is now quelled with the processed and prepackaged images of television, movies, and video games. Are we unwittingly engaging the services of professional dreamers to do our dreaming for us?

Complement this with the excessive consumption of alcohol, tranquilizers, and sleeping pills, all of which also suppress dreaming, and you have an unrecognized public and spiritual health hazard that is wreaking havoc with our consciousness and exacerbating our night blindness.

Disordered Awakening

For most of us, night ends much like it begins—mindlessly. Our disregard for dusk and darkness is complemented by a similar posture toward dawn and daybreak. Morning in modern times has little to do with the rising of the sun and the advent of the day's new light. It is now complicated by symptoms of sleep and dream deprivation, substance and sleeping pill hangovers, a frenetic groping for counterfeit energy, and, of course, another rush hour.

Most Americans are too chronically sleep deprived to awaken without an alarm. By definition, an alarm signals some kind of danger. Millions of us routinely hit our snooze buttons to steal a few extra moments of desperately needed sleep on most weekday mornings. Then there's the task of dragging a resistant body out of bed, followed by the ultimate morning challenge, that of "coming to." The majority of us cannot awaken without a hearty hit of caffeine. When we finally do begin to come to, we are typically more concerned with the morning news than with the natural newness of morning.

We are most vulnerable in the morning. Complex changes in body and mind occur as we approach awakening. Our melatonin levels have peaked, cortisol is on the rise, our body temperature has bottomed out, and our psyches are deeply immersed in dreams. It is indeed darkest before the dawn. Like birth, morning awakening is a time of a tricky biological and psychological transition as well as a time of unique sacred possibility.

In actuality, we do not awaken in the morning from sleep but from our dreams. Unfortunately, we usually dismiss this critical transitional process—this hybrid state of dreaming and waking—by demeaning it as grogginess. In doing so, we forgo an exceptional opportunity to access an extraordinary state of consciousness.

How we awaken in the morning establishes a trajectory that powerfully influences the quality of our day. It sets both a direction and a pace for the day, which is typically fast, driven, and overly industrious. Modern morning routines have replaced more traditional, spiritual morning rituals that graciously greet the new day. Less hurried cultures continue to celebrate the dawn with prayer, meditation, and setting conscious intentions for the day.

During the first night of a visit to Jerusalem's Old City, an ancient neighborhood composed of different religious sects, I was jolted from my jet-lagged slumber by the broadcast of predawn Muslim prayers. I grumbled, turned, and fell back asleep, only to be roused again just moments later by the loud murmur of Jewish morning services. Frustrated, I managed to return to sleep once again, only to be awakened a third time by the clang of Christian church bells echoing down the old narrow alleyways. Different as each of these sects' approaches to morning are, they share a common theme of intentional and sacred awakening. In contrast to the sounds of modern mornings—the clamor of commuter trains and buses, congested traffic, growling garbage trucks, and construction down the street—these more traditional approaches reflect the sacred potential at the start of each new day.

The vast majority of us today rarely witness dawn or a sunrise. We have forgotten the wonder of a gradual awakening to soft light and bird songs. Instead, millions of us awaken each morning unrefreshed, underslept, hung over, unhappy, and somewhat dazed— simply not ready to start another day. Such mindless morning awakenings keep resetting tired old agendas and trajectories for brand-new days. Rather than celebrate morning, many people struggle through or even curse its arrival. There may now be new truth in the old saying, "The reason most people get up in the morning is that they didn't die in their sleep." Like poor sleepers who unknowingly never really venture into deep sleep, many of us are poor risers who struggle even more than we know with becoming fully awake.

Disordered Waking

Beyond being chronically sleep and dream deprived, we are also considerably wake deprived. What many of us consider normal waking is not. Our failure to descend deeply into sleep and dreams compromises our ability to ascend fully into the waking world. The once naturally robust peaks and valleys of our circadian cycles are in danger of flatlining. Unfortunately, millions of us have habituated to waking life in a pernicious mental *daze*.

Numerous studies suggest that the chronic sleep and dream loss by night contaminates the quality of our wakefulness by day. "Everything looks better after a good night's sleep," says a Chinese proverb. No doubt the opposite is also true. Chronic poor sleep distorts our perception and negatively affects our mood, exacerbating life's waking challenges. Sleep and dream debt can leave us disoriented, depressed, and, as we will see, even dangerous. Our mental daze is further complicated by our peculiar tendency to avoid natural daylight.

Despite evidence suggesting that sunlight is naturally stimulating, emotionally uplifting, and potentially healing, we spend the bulk of our waking days indoors. When the sun sets, we usually turn on lights and remain indoors. When it becomes light outside, however, we again turn on lights and remain indoors. Compared to dusk and night, indoor lighting is bright and overstimulating. But in contrast to natural daylight, even on cloudy days, indoor light is relatively dim and understimulating. The average American adult gets about one hour of natural outdoor light exposure each day. Considering that this average figure accounts for people like gardeners, golfers, construction workers, and others who are routinely outside, it highlights our strange resistance to solar consciousness.

Our loss of sleep and dreaming's nightly restoration coupled with this lack of natural daytime stimulation leaves us chronically depleted. Sleepiness and fatigue are among the most common complaints heard by primary care physicians. We compensate for and mask our depletion with counterfeit energies that spike sharply but crash precipitously, encouraging a vicious cycle of continued use. In the end, this pattern only serves to exacerbate our chronic mental daze and reinforce our denial of it.

me!

The emperor has no doze. The widespread cultural and personal denial of our mental daze may be the greatest consensual pretense of our times. We know that the emperor is severely sleep and dream deprived. And we strongly suspect that he is using—that is, he is doing something to mask his waking daze. But out of blind regard for empirical authority, we remain in cahoots with the charade. One cannot help but wonder if this common, collective daze we call waking might not function like Aldous Huxley's "soma," serving to sedate the masses, thereby enabling them to better cope with the untenable demands of their driven lives.

Healing Darkness

With the gradual erosion of night we witness a corresponding erosion of health and consciousness. The damage to our sleep, dreams, and waking consciousness is both subtle and glaring. It is subtle because it has evolved gradually, slowly, quietly over a number of generations, establishing itself as the norm. And it is glaring because when we are willing to step back out of the current of mass mentality, we quickly realize how far we have drifted from our nature, and how damaging to both body and mind this is.

I believe we may suffer from a darkness deficiency. Recent findings suggest that there may be beneficial effects associated with time awake in darkened space. Just as light stimulates the release of serotonin, which energizes us, darkness encourages the production of melatonin, the key neurohormone in our night biology, sleep, and dreams. Excessive light at night along with other features of modern life conversely inhibit melatonin, dampening the positive effects of darkness.

Our very consciousness is in need of repair. Like the attention deficit world we live in, it is scattered—segregated, even fragmented. Sleep and dreams are sharply set apart from waking, although fragments of these states now cut and bleed into one another. We see an epidemic of wakefulness intruding into our sleep and dreams as insomnia. The resulting sleep and dream debt seeps back into our wakefulness as the dangerous mental smog of daze. We mistake the jittery buzz of counterfeit energies for natural vitality. Half-awake in our sleep and half-asleep in our waking, we are never completely at rest and seldom fully conscious.

Despite years of well-intended effort on the part of groups like the National Sleep Foundation and the American Academy of Sleep Medicine to address our night blindness, matters are getting worse. Like the night-blinded culture they represent, these organizations routinely fail to acknowledge the critical role of personal and spiritual dimensions of night. They fail to acknowledge night consciousness. Philosophically, they approach the evaluation and treatment of our damaged nights by illuminating them with the light of ordinary waking understanding. This is akin to trying explore darkness using a flashlight. It is the night blind leading the night blind. We will heal night only when we are willing to understand it on its own dark terms.

Night is the shadow of the Earth. It is as nature intended, dark. And unsettling. Since darkness deprives us of vision, our primary means of orienting to and managing the outer world, it dissolves essential aspects of our social, extraverted selves. Most of us are probably less afraid of the dark per se, but more frightened of what darkness might reveal. Darkness drives us inward where we are confronted with disowned aspects of our psychological selves, our own *shadow*. Our fear of darkness is best understood in terms

Loss will.

of what Carl Jung first called "shadow." I believe that night is a natural medium for shadow work.

Denied Emotions

Shadow is the internal representation of darkness, the disowned murky aspects of ourselves, all that we wish not to be. So much of what we necessarily rebuff throughout our driven days gets relegated to night. Night becomes a repository for all that we deny, suppress, and project outward over the course of waking consciousness. Like a self-storage space packed to capacity, this dark matter bulges and breaks out when our watchman dares to rest or sleep.

Sprouting under the cover of darkness like mushrooms from dirt, our shadows emerge naturally by night. They draw mysterious elements of the earth upward, offering us a strange kind of sustenance, a foreign fare that leaves us sharply ambivalent. We are most willing to flirt with images of darkness so long as they are sanitized and depersonalized by various forms of media. But flirtation is not a relationship. I believe that our reluctance to deal directly with our essential fear of darkness is the major impediment to our rapprochement with night, sleep, and dreams. Accessing the healing power of night requires that we engage in shadow work. And we will get dirty.

Healing Night is about becoming nightminded. Using an approach I call *nocturnal lucidity*, it is about courageously extending our awareness into arenas we believe lie outside of our awareness. It is a way of seeing in the dark.

Creats a space for more understanding.

Lucidity is the primary healing approach used in this book. Going beyond its most common association with dreaming, we will see that lucidity is a valuable way of approaching all aspects of night consciousness. If mindfulness is about becoming more aware of subtle daytime waking experiences, lucidity is a mindfulness of night.

With our worldly eyes closed, but with the mind's eye open, we step intentionally into a dark space but refrain from flipping on the lights. The mind's eye dilates, and our inner vision gradually acclimates to a delicate glow that backlights the night, revealing sacred mysteries concealed in the shadows.

⌒ 2

The Rhythm of Rest

For everything there is a season,
and a time for every purpose under heaven.

—ECCLESIASTES

TOM WAS A DRIVEN, THIRTY-TWO-YEAR-OLD MALE who vehemently defended his blind devotion to work, productivity, and achievement. He was exceptionally energetic, industrious, and creative but almost mechanical in his relentless pursuit of success. Tom's unchecked drive often obscured his regard for his own basic, personal needs. He did not eat, sleep, or care for himself or his family well. His wife and children were among the casualties of his obstinate drive.

Through extended periods of his life, Tom worked at his projects with an almost manic pace. During such marathon sessions he chain-smoked cigars, drank heavily, and slept little. Over the years he became severely dependent on alcohol and, eventually, morphine to help him slow down and sleep. Tom was outspoken about his disregard for sleep. Sleeping more than three hours a night, he believed, was a sign of being lazy and indolent. "Sleep," he said, "is like a drug. Take too much at a time and it makes you dopey. You lose time and opportunities."

Tom was Tom Edison, Thomas Alva Edison, the inventor of the electric light bulb.

It was 1879 and the Industrial Revolution was sweeping across the Western world with an almost religious zeal. The machine, which held the promise of social and economic salvation, was emerging as a role model. Edison's deepest desire was to illuminate the night, enabling people to operate 24/7—like machines. And his light bulb was born of this kind of mechanically inspired, sleep-deprived, and substance-driven industrial marathon. What an apt beginning for what electric lighting would help bring to our world—a mechanically inspired, sleep-deprived, and substance-driven industrial marathon we call life.

Edison's victory over night symbolized a significant turning point in culture's domination of nature. In the decades to follow, excessive LAN (light at night) would significantly erode our experience of dusk, darkness, and dawn. By dampening our awareness of the essential pulse of day and night, of light and darkness, LAN has undermined our relationship to life's fundamental rhythmicity. Nature's rhythmic definition of our lives would give way to culture's relentless drive, resulting in a widespread, pernicious *dysrhythmia*. As we will see, dysrhythmic life patterns impair our capacity for rest and resonance—the basic ways in which we relate to the world and one another, and the quality of our sleep, dreams, and awakening. A major factor in our night blindness, our loss of life's natural rhythms has radically transformed culture and consciousness.

It was as if we had suddenly come of age with the advent of electric lighting. Mother Nature could no longer insist that we go to bed at her designated hour. Like impetuous adolescents we could now claim the freedom to delay, limit, and even forgo rest and sleep. And we do. For many, life today is informed by the same kind of incessant drive evident in Edison's work and times. As reflected in our curious reverence for marathon events, Guinness world endurance records, planes that refuel without landing, heroes with robotic features, and the now nearly mythic Energizer Bunny, we are a culture enamored with people and things that can keeping going, and going, and going . . . These are things that do not need to rest and, consequently, have little sensitivity to natural rhythms.

Before the advent of electric night lighting, the natural order of life—poetically reflected in the Old Testament's Ecclesiastes, was still fundamentally rhythmic. There was *a season and a time for every purpose*. A gentle but firm sense of rhythm framed and structured daily life, activity, and consciousness. With familiar and comforting arms, Mother Nature gently cradled and steadily rocked us. In the decades that followed, however, nature's rhythmic definition of our lives gave way to culture's relentless drive. Today, it seems more like there is *a reason and a purpose for every time*.

The rocking chair was once a classic symbol of American leisure. In Norman Rockwell–era images of the Sunday afternoon gathering on the front porch, family and friends would sit rocking, resting, and relating. Our traditional regard for the rocking chair has been displaced by a soaring reverence for the rocket ship. Excessive LAN has ignited a powerful cultural thrust that has displaced nature's rhythm of activity and rest. Incessant drive has become the default cadence of contemporary life. We are off our rockers, restless, and dysrhythmic.

Rhythms

I have vivid memories of watching my children watching *Sesame Street* when they were young. Curiously, they rejoiced in viewing what I thought were frequent and needless repetitions of various segments in the same show. "I'm going to paint a seven," said some silly guy in a funny hat who then proceeded to paint a large seven. A few short moments later, same scene, same guy, same silly hat, and same line, "I'm going to paint a seven." And again and again. My children loved it, and many other similar routines as well. As much as they are attracted to novelty, we know that children are also drawn to repetition, regularity, and routine. "Again, Daddy. Again. Again . . ." Children love rhythms.

From the oscillation of atomic particles to the swirl of galaxies, from brain waves to the beat of the heart, and from the tempo of day and night to the seasons of the sun, rhythms literally rule our world. And they regulate us. From merry-go-rounds to rock and roll, from personal routines and religious rituals to standard operating procedures, rhythms provide a structure for virtually all aspects of life. In the course of our daily lives, rhythms serve as clocks and calendars, as metronomes and baselines, telling us when it is and, consequently, what to do. Rhythms tell us when to breathe, eat, mate, when to be active, and when to rest. And they tell us when to sleep, dream, and awaken. Science is just beginning to discover what sacred traditions have known all along—rhythms are ubiquitous, powerful, and healing.

Rhythms have always had a central place in spiritual thought and practices around the world. Rhythmic procedures are central to most approaches to meditation, prayer, yoga, holiday celebrations, and other religious and spiritual rituals.

The Greek gods of antiquity provided a cosmic framework for rhythmic order in natural and human affairs. A key feature of mythology, in fact, is the impact of such overarching celestial influences on daily, mundane human life.

Nyx, the primordial goddess of night, emerged early in the evolution of the Greek pantheon. Among the most influential of divine beings, her progeny included the gods and goddesses of sleep, dreams, daytime, and even death. Nyx's power was evident not only in her progeny but also in her grand responsibility to deliver and manage night. Like other major gods and goddesses, she provided an important comforting sense of predictability and reliability. Although clocks as we know them were not yet invented, we might say she was like clockwork. We might think of her as a fundamental expression of regularity—a term that today conjures up more mundane associations with bowel habits and laxatives. Even our language is inadequate to describe the grandeur of rhythmicity. The Chinese, however, do have such a language.

The familiar *yin-yang* symbol reminds us of the ubiquity of rhythms throughout the universe. Consisting of a black and a white tear-shaped wave enclosed in a circle, the yin-yang suggests that the entire universe is governed by a single, unifying rhythmic principle. The white wave, or *yang*, represents the principles of the masculine, including the sun, day, light, activation, and drive, while the black wave, or *yin*, symbolizes the principles of the feminine, including the moon, night, darkness, rest, and receptivity. Chinese philosophy teaches that all things in the universe can be understood in terms of the rhythmic interaction and balance between these two opposite but complementary forces. Suggestive of perpetual rotation, the yin-yang conveys a sense that all things will eventually transform into their opposites. Chinese medicine continues to use the philosophy and language of the yin-yang, offering a deep regard for the role of rhythmicity in life and health. As symbol and language, the yin-yang elegantly depicts the rhythmic essence of all things as well as the essence of all rhythmic processes.

Whether at cosmic, cultural, or consciousness levels, rhythms can be thought of as patterns that underlie the expression, movement, or flow of energy. Like the yin-yang, science conceives of energy in terms of waves, which, like ocean waves, can vary greatly in their magnitude and motion. These variations produce the unique signature of rhythms. Whether it is the "energy" of a culture, an individual, or a drop of water, there are distinctive qualities about all things that are reflected in their rhythmic signatures.

Just as ocean waves are contained within the larger rhythmic structure of the tide, there are lower- and higher-order rhythms. It is useful to think of ourselves as complex, interactive energy systems defined by the rhythmic activities of the body and mind—of hormones, circulation, digestion, brain waves, and states of consciousness, for example. At the same time, we are embedded in larger social, cultural, environmental, and cosmic energy systems that exert powerful influences over us. We depend on smaller, lower-order rhythmic patterns "below" in the form of our biology, and "above" us in the form of our cosmology.

Who we are involves a complex interaction of higher and lower wave patterns: our culture, family and friends, the environment, on one hand, and our biology, brains, and biochemistry, on the other. When in balance, this represents the marriage of the sun and moon, of heaven and earth, yin and yang. In modern life, however, our higher-order rhythmic influences are less about the natural environment and much more about culture. Although cultural rhythmic patterns can be beautifully expressed in the arts—especially social ritual, music, and dance—the overriding signatures of modern culture are erratic, staccato, hurried, and essentially dysrhythmic. Because they do not allow for sufficient rest, we might say that these patterns are excessively yang, or insufficient in yin.

More specifically, lower-order bodily rhythms that influence our energies and needs for rest are easily overridden by higher-order cultural rhythms that dictate occupational and recreation schedules. Such cultural influences override human nature in large part by buffering signals from the natural environment.

Old Faithful is the best-known geyser in Yellowstone National Park, deriving its name from the fact that it erupts in average periods of about ninety minutes with great regularity. Rhythms provide order, something we can have faith in. Whether we believe this order is scientific or spiritual, benign or kind, conscious or mechanical, rhythms can remind us of the presence of a higher order or greater power in our lives. As we will see, healing our night consciousness requires that we acknowledge and consciously relate to such a higher order, an order that is higher even than culture.

Living with and within a conscious sense of rhythm is comforting and healing. Research has confirmed that people and animals are comforted by repetitive rhythmic or stereotypic behavior. Whether through the rocking of a rocking chair or the rock in "rock and roll," rhythmicity elicits a soothing neurochemical response in the brain. Routines, standard operating procedures, and temporal structures are all about rhythm. Obviously, rhythm is the foundation of music, dance, and all forms of ritual. It also lies at the core of our very life in the form of the breath.

Breathing may be the most fundamental expression of rhythmicity in human life. Some believe that the ancient Hebrew name of God, *Yahweh,* was derived from the sound of a full breath flowing in and out of the mouth. Breathing is the only physiological function that can operate on both completely conscious and completely unconscious levels. In this way, it seems to serve as an essential bridge between consciousness and unconsciousness—between yang and yin. Changes in breathing patterns are known to be associated with changes in consciousness. More shallow and rapid breathing is characteristic of more aroused states, while deeper and slower breathing is associated with relaxation, meditative states, and sleep. Breathing connects the lower-order rhythms of our biology with the higher-order rhythms of consciousness.

Rhythms of Consciousness

Like the yin-yang, our planet is always half illuminated, half dark. The rotation of the earth spins each hemisphere through daily cycles of light and dark. This pattern has become deeply imprinted on our biology in the form of an internal biological clock. Also known as a circadian (from *circa*, meaning "about," and *dies*, meaning "day") pacemaker, this small bundle of cells situated near the center of the brain tells us when it is—when to be active and when to rest, when to wake and when to sleep. Our very consciousness, that is, our basic sleep-dream-wake cycle, is circadian in nature, born of and structured by nature's cycles of light and darkness.

Modern medicine is just discovering the powerful role of circadian rhythms in maintaining mental and physical health. Biology recapitulates cosmology. Circadian rhythms mete out a basic temporal framework for our biology, including our endocrine, immune, cardiovascular, digestive, and central nervous system functions. They strongly influence states of arousal, our performance, as well as our need for food and drink. These personal rhythms are derived from and designed to run in sync with much larger cosmic rhythms.

Although circadian rhythms are the primary baseline in the song of life on Earth, they are just one part of a complex symphony that also incorporates many other rhythmic lines. *Infradian* rhythms refer to cyclic patterns that are longer than a day. These include the familiar examples of reproductive and menstrual cycles as well as other complex developmental changes in our biology and behavior.

Of greater relevance to understanding consciousness, including sleeping, dreaming, and waking, are *ultradian* rhythms. Ultradian rhythms refer to cyclic patterns that recur in periods of less than a day. Heart rate, respiration, and brain waves are examples of relatively fast ultradian rhythms since they occur numerous times daily. Sometimes referred to as nature's hour, primary ultradian rhythms have an average period of about ninety minutes. Also known as *basic rest and activity cycles,* or BRAC, these rhythms occur throughout the day and night providing a structure for rhythmic shifts in our consciousness. As the name *BRAC* implies, the fundamental structure of our consciousness is activity and rest—yang and yin.

Throughout the waking day, approximately seventy minutes of each ninety-minute BRAC period is characterized by ordinary waking consciousness. We are active, attentive, focused, and potentially productive. The last twenty minutes or so of each BRAC period, however, involves a shift to a more expansive and diffused kind of consciousness. It calls for a break from ordinary activity, drawing us into a dream-like realm, into imagination. It calls for rest. As we will see in our discussion of waking, the daytime influence of BRAC is subtle, and, not surprisingly, its rest component is frequently overridden by our incessant drive. Occupational law requires that we take fifteen-minute "coffee breaks" from work every few hours. Natural law is more lenient, encouraging us to take more frequent, twenty-minute breaks.

The Rhythm of Night Consciousness

By night, BRAC becomes the procedural framework for our *sleep architecture,* the rhythmic structure of our sleep and dream cycles. Usually depicted in terms of jagged lines representing brain wave activity, sleep architecture is actually less a structure and more a process. Each ninety-minute ultradian sleep cycle is made up of two discrete kinds of consciousness, sleeping and dreaming. We normally spend more of the first half of the night in actual sleep, whereas dreaming, or REM, becomes more prominent in the second half of the night.

Specific states of consciousness—sleeping, dreaming, and waking—are measured in terms of brain waves, which are complex rhythmic patterns of electrical energy emitted by brain activity.

Also known as electroencephalography, or EEG, brain waves are defined in terms of their speed or frequency in cycles per second (Hz). Brain waves create distinct signatures that reflect subtle gradations of waking, sleeping, and dreaming states.

The four major brain wave patterns are *beta, alpha, theta,* and *delta* waves. Normal waking consciousness in which our attention is focused primarily on the outer world is dominated by beta waves, which have a frequency of fourteen cycles per second or greater. Alpha waves, defined by frequencies of eight to thirteen cycles per second, are associated with a relaxed waking state. With sensory awareness withdrawn from the outer world, slower theta waves, ranging from four to seven cycles per second, are associated with deeply relaxed waking states such as meditation as well as with lighter sleep. Finally, deep and relatively quiescent delta waves, which range from five to three cycles per second, are characteristic of exceptional states of serenity seen in advanced meditation practices and are also associated with our deepest sleep.

In practical terms, EEG, or brain wave patterns, are often mixed and overlapping, resulting in various gradations and hybrid states of consciousness. It is interesting to note, for example, that EEG patterns characteristic of sleep can also occur during very restful waking states. Likewise, dreaming, as well as the transitions between waking and sleeping, typically reflect a mix of waking and sleeping EEG activity.

Sleep itself is made up of four continuous, deepening stages that are defined by specific ranges of brain wave activity. The transition from waking to sleep, referred to as Stage 1 or *threshold* sleep, is associated with a mix of waking beta waves and relaxed waking alpha waves. By convention, formal sleep onset occurs in Stage 2 sleep and involves a mix of slower alpha and theta waves. Stage 3 and Stage 4 sleep, collectively referred to as *deep sleep* or *slow wave* sleep, are characterized by theta and delta waves. Each ultradian sleep cycle normally includes a sequence of sleep stages followed by a period of dreaming, or REM, sleep.

The quality and proportion of time we spend in various sleep stages and dreaming can vary widely with age and health. In our world, sleeping and dreaming too often degrade as a result of our aging, our dependence on substances and medications, and our devaluing night consciousness. By midlife, the majority of Americans experience little, if any, deep sleep as well as significantly diminished dreaming. I believe that these changes are associated with a pernicious breakdown of our natural rhythms.

Resonance

In 1665, Christian Huygens, a Dutch astronomer and inventor of the pendulum clock, observed a curious phenomenon. Two of the larger clocks in his workshop began to beat in unison. He found that no matter how they might be stopped, started, or disrupted, they returned to a synchronized pattern of oscillation. At the risk of being excessively anthropomorphic, we might say they began going together.

Love →

There is a natural, ubiquitous, and powerful innate tendency in all things, living and otherwise, to "go together,"—to synchronize their rhythmic activity. The complex rhythmic signatures that make up all things will resonate, harmonize, or, in more technical terms, *entrain* with one another when they are in proximity. Groups of fireflies blink synchronously, individual cardiac pacemaker cells maintain a steady heartbeat, and women who share living space report that their menstrual cycles synchronize. Gary Schwartz and Linda Russek, my colleagues at the University of Arizona, found that heart and brain rhythms of people sitting quietly together would also synchronize. In all of these examples, the synchronization of separate oscillators, or "clocks," allows for a kind of coordinated or collective behavior to emerge—a coming together.

I prefer to think of this universal tendency toward the synchronization of independent rhythms in general terms of *resonance*. Depending on their receptivity, individual cells, animals, people, events, and virtually all other things can resonate with and potentially influence one another's rhythms. *Resonance is the essential process underlying all relating.* What we resonate with, consciously or unconsciously, profoundly shapes our experience and behavior. It determines the essential tempo of our lives, including the complex rhythmic patterns of our daily activities and nightly rest. Resonance mediates our relationship with nature's circadian rhythms as well as our connection with cultural forces. It is about the interaction, coordination, and synchronization of life's complex clocks.

The specific kind of resonance that affects our sleep, dreaming, and waking patterns is referred to as *entrainment*. Just as it sounds, the notion of entraining is associated with the idea of boarding and riding a train. When we ride a train, it carries us along at its own rhythmic pace; we go with or become entrained to it. Most of us are unknowingly carried along throughout our daily lives by various conceptual trains. These trains do not take us from place to place but from time to time. We entrain with the movement, activity, energy, and pace around us. The tempos of our surroundings, workplace, community, and social environment imbue a sense of time into our lives. They tell us when to get up and when to go to bed, when to work and when to sleep, when to be active and when to rest. Because they provide us with a sense of time, they are referred to as *zeitgebers*—from the German, "time-givers."

There are three types of zeitgebers that influence our circadian and ultradian rhythms: personal, natural, and cultural clocks. Our personal clocks, also known as our body clocks, reflect our inner and biological sense of time. Natural time, of course, is defined by rhythmic changes in nature, primarily through the ebb and flow of light and darkness. And cultural time, in much of our world, is about the rapid paced rhythm of overly industrious life. Ultimately, our personal sense of time is determined by the resonance between our inner clock—our personal and biological zeitgebers—and our outer clock—defined to varying degrees by culture or nature. The train most of us ride each day is a cultural express.

Entrainment requires a connection between two or more zeitgebers that is usually determined by proximity. Huygens's clocks were close by, in the same workshop. Huygens also noticed that larger pendulum clocks seemed to impose their rhythmic pattern on smaller ones. Larger, more powerful rhythmic forces will entrain smaller, less powerful ones. Entrainment, then, also depends on the potency of and our receptivity to particular zeitgebers. Historically, zeitgebers were largely natural. In nature, the ebb and flow of light and dark signaled the primary temporal frameworks of life. Today, the larger, more potent, and most proximal zeitgebers derived from culture override nature's rhythmic signature.

Dysrhythmias

A meaningful understanding of modern patterns of sleeping, dreaming, and awakening requires that we consider them in the context of the dysrhythmic culture that birthed and sustains them. Impossible demands of our work, family, and social lives routinely throw the majority of Americans out of sync with nature's circadian rhythms. The overriding rhythmic structure of modern life is irregular, hurried, staccato, and relentless. Speeding is the most common infraction of the law. We are "jet-setters" living in the "fast lane," caught up in the "rat race," and sick with "hurry sickness." We suffer from a collective tachycardia, a rapid, runaway cultural heartbeat. As the symphonic rhythms of nature, including human nature, are persistently overridden, we become deeply entrained with the dysrhythmic cacophony of modern culture.

A standard day is no longer defined by nature's circadian timing but by culture's artificial time. Our experiences and behaviors are structured by artificial zeitgebers—tics and tocks, bells, beeps, buzzes, sirens, horns, and chimes. It is no longer the crow of the cock, but the buzz of the alarm clock that defines the arrival of morning. And at the other end, in lieu of Nyx, Letterman, Leno, and the late news define the onset of night. Such culture-driven cues override natural zeitgebers like dusk and dawn, hunger and satiety, sleepiness and wakefulness. We get up and go to bed when cultural time, not natural timing, dictates. And we usually eat, work, exercise, rest, and generally live in response to these artificial zeitgebers—a kind of cultured time.

Caught between the frequently conflicting messages of personal, natural, and cultural clocks, we often do not really know exactly "when" it is. We live in a kind of temporal disorientation, not clearly knowing when to sleep, dream, or awaken.

Our subjective sense of night, that is, our personal clock's designation about when we should be asleep, is referred to as our *sleep phase*. Unfortunately, our sleep phase can be out of sync with the objective, cultural clock's designation of our sleep schedule. Such desynchrony can result in *sleep phase disorders*, which are potent factors in various types of insomnia. In *advanced sleep phase*, more common as we age, our personal clocks run fast, believing it is bedtime some hours before the outer clock does. Because one's rising time is also advanced, an advanced sleep phase is frequently associated with very early morning awakenings and difficulty returning to sleep. The converse is true with *delayed sleep phase*, which is quite common in adolescence. With this condition our personal clocks run slow, insisting that bed and rising times occur a few hours later than the outer clock suggests. Trying to get to sleep before our personal clock believes it is bedtime is a common cause of sleep onset insomnia. And needing to awaken before our personal clock believes it is morning can leave us excessively sleepy upon arising.

In addition to sleep phase disorders, dysrhythmias are associated with other common conditions such as jet lag, shift work, and irregular sleep-wake schedules. Beyond their deleterious impact on sleep and dreams, many studies confirm that circadian dysrhythmias are associated with significant increases in depression, chronic illness, and mortality. I believe that dysrhythmias also influence our health, happiness, and spirituality in other ways that we are just beginning to discover. Dysrhythmias are ultimately the result of our incessant drive, which suppresses the rest phase of our BRAC. Why are we so driven to forgo rest?

Rest

"Let me tell you something, Doc. I've been on the high road for years and never had to downshift before. Everybody's telling me I need to slow, but I don't see a red light anywhere. Nobody wins by dawdling in the pit stop, you know." Rod, a successful middle-aged businessman, was a new client whose focus was so insular that it took two or three jabs on my part to derail his stream of consciousness and join the conversation.

"So, Rod . . . excuse me. Uh, let me just ask . . . what brings you in?" I squeezed in one of my usual openings for new clients at the health resort where I consulted.

"Oh . . . uh . . ." Rod managed a thoughtful pause, "Well, Doc, I think what I really need is a tune-up."

Vague as it is, asking for a tune-up is a rather common, socially acceptable, and emotionally accessible avenue to a psychological consult. It is certainly preferable to having to admit that one feels anxious or depressed, or that one's spouse thinks one is crazy. And like many other clients, Rod seemed to believe that the term *tune-up* was a kind of definitive diagnostic statement for which I could now offer a clinically astute prescription.

A *tune-up*, I mused. Though I had heard this phrase many times before in the same context, it suddenly caught my attention in a new way. The term, obviously derived from automobile maintenance, seemed to fit. As I got to know him better, it became apparent that Rod was, indeed, imbued with the spirit of a car.

Over the years, I have heard numerous variations on this self-as-automobile theme from hundreds of people. A middle-aged woman who worked tirelessly at managing family problems told me she needed to learn how to *apply the brakes*. A burned-out Wall Street broker told me he needed to *recharge his batteries*. A young athlete recovering from an injury wanted to *get back into gear*. An elderly man with a chronic medical condition wanted a *green light* from his doctor. Still another executive set a goal of *refueling*. And others, many others, wanted to *shift gears,* get a *jump-start,* or get a *grip on the wheel*. In addition to psychological "tune-ups," many of these people also sought *bodywork*. And, of course, a routine part of a basic health assessment includes getting one's *oil* (cholesterol) *checked*.

Whether we acknowledge it or not, many of us are simply *driven*.

Much has been written about America's love affair with cars, but I had never considered how deeply this identification had rooted itself in our psyches. Anthropologists have long recognized a universal tendency, most clearly seen in indigenous cultures, to identify with the spirit of things like rivers, the moon, or, most commonly, animals. Identification with animals can evoke specific desirable qualities—courage, perspective, and intelligence, for example. These are usually identifications with living or natural things, things that experience rhythms of activity and rest, of waking and sleeping. Cars are mechanisms, machines. Theoretically, short of running out of gas and mechanical breakdown, they can just keep on going and going.

Why do we struggle so with rest? *True rest can result in the opportunistic emergence of suppressed psychological material.* Swept up by industrial drive, I believe we often fail to even acknowledge our need for rest because we fear slowing down and stopping. As long as we maintain a healthy clip, we prevent all that stuff swept into the night repository from rising into consciousness. If we do hit the brakes, unwanted thoughts and feelings stashed in the back of our vehicle might come flying forward. All the shadowy stuff we have been too busy to deal with, the accumulated hurts, fears, confusions, as well as all of our old unresolved personal issues threaten to overtake us if we dare to slow or stop.

"Nothing is so intolerable to man as being fully at rest," said Blaise Pascal. Too often, we develop an aversive reaction to the unexpected and unwanted upsurge of psychological material, blaming slowing down for the discomfort that emerges. We attribute this discomfort to the call of unfinished chores, work, or other activities. Resuming activity diverts attention from our discomfort and reinforces the mistaken sense that we felt bad either because we were resting or because we simply should have kept moving. Incessant activity can also conceal underlying mood disturbances, especially depression, that threaten to surface if we do not remain vigilant.

I have found that many people frequently deny, distort, or become confused about the call to rest—about their subjective experience of "tiredness." The word *tired* can actually refer to a number of different experiences that are usually not well differentiated. In addition to its reference to emotional states like sadness and frustration (as in *I'm so tired of that*), tiredness refers to the experiences of sleepiness and fatigue.

Although they frequently overlap, sleepiness and fatigue are distinctly different states that call for different responses. Sleepiness, which obviously results from inadequate sleep, is associated with heavy eyelids and a heavy head. When we are sleepy, our attentiveness or sensory connection to the world is withdrawn. Obviously, sleepiness signals a need for sleep. In contrast, fatigue refers to physical exhaustion or muscular depletion usually experienced as a heavy or droopy body. Our capacity to respond to or express ourselves in the world is diminished. In contrast to sleepiness, I believe that fatigue is more accurately understood as a need to rest.

Severe and debilitating forms of fatigue are usually symptomatic of physical or emotional illness. We might think of the more ordinary experience of fatigue as a signal to shift from activity to the rest phase of our BRAC. As we will see in our discussion of dreaming, fatigue may actually be symptomatic of a need to dream.

Role modeling the incessant drive of adults, we learn very young not to acknowledge or trust feelings of sleepiness or fatigue. Unless done within the tight constraints of social norms, public displays of rest are suspect and associated with being infirm, ill, or otherwise out of it. As a reflection of mistrust of their subjective experience, many people literally check the time to determine whether they need to rest. In our discussion of waking, we will consider the common error of confusing a genuine need for rest with a need for counterfeit energy.

When we finally do acknowledge our need to rest, we often confuse genuine rest with activity, recreation, and substance use. After I repeatedly encouraged my friend Annette to get more rest, she sent me a note describing her sincere attempt to do so:

> I had been going nonstop for the past week or so, and last night was my first night home. So what did I do? I got into bed to watch a good TV movie with lots of propped up pillows, wine, chocolate, and a magazine for the commercials.

Annette's attempt at rest reflects some common, yet erroneous notions that confuse rest with recreation, stimulation, and the use of substances. Annette recognized that she was worn down and decided to be good to herself by resting. She did manage to get physically comfortable, an important ingredient in rest. But in addition to consuming a sugary snack and alcohol, Annette also confused "rest" with entertainment and incessant stimulation. *A magazine for the commercials.*

For many, the thought of rest conjures images of tennis, golf, swimming, hiking, biking, or other athletic activities. For others, it is a good book, magazine, or movie. I certainly have no argument with exercise or entertainment of this sort and frequently recommend them to my patients. But are they truly restful, or just a substitution of other activity?

For some, being tired has become a cue to alter one's consciousness with alcohol or other substances. The need to rest conjures thoughts of a glass of wine, a cold beer, a martini. For others, rest is about rolling a joint or taking a hit of a pipe. Altering one's consciousness with substances as a means of resting is a complex social and health issue. Though the deeper intention beneath getting high may actually be a positive desire to slow down and rest, this strategy usually backfires. Using substances, or food for that matter, with the primary intention of escaping, avoiding, or denying personal issues is not conducive to true rest.

If rest is not about activity, recreation, or a substance-driven escape, then what is it? Basic rest and activity cycles (BRAC) remind us that rest is the counterpoint to activity. It is not an activity per se, not about being productive or utilitarian. Common methods of rest include meditation, prayer, and yoga. Or just sitting. Sitting on the porch, sitting quietly, rocking, lying on the couch, strolling in a garden. Sometimes being at rest might look like being depressed, offensive to the workaholic in each of us. One of my colleagues hung a poster to remind him to rest in his busy medical office. It was the image of a smiling chimpanzee sitting with feet on a desk and arms behind his head. The caption beneath read "Sometimes I sits and think—and sometimes I just sits."

I think of true rest as the waking expression of night consciousness—a kind of low-grade, or subliminal, waking sleep and dream state. Associated with mixed EEG patterns such as alpha, theta, and even delta states, rest is a kind of slow-wave waking. As we proceed, we will see that rest is an essential prerequisite to healthy sleep and dreams, to natural night consciousness. And like night, rest has important healing and spiritual dimensions.

Rest is healing. Rest is a universal and critical ingredient in virtually all approaches to healing. We are almost always advised to get bed rest when we are ill. Rest is essential for emotional healing as well. Psychologists are forever telling people to "relax"—a two-syllable word for rest. As we will see, I believe that rest is a largely overlooked treatment for depression.

While images of hell are usually characterized by endless toil, images of heaven from around the world are associated with leisure and rest. Most spiritual techniques and practices are also restful or informed by a resting posture. Meditation, yoga, tai chi, and prayer are usually practiced in a mindful, restful manner. In discussing prayer with many of my patients over the years, I was surprised to find that while listening for divine guidance, they frequently heard variations of the same answer: rest. Rest, like sleep, is a behavioral expression of faith. When we rest, we do so because we believe that all is or will be in order.

For many of us, when we finally do rest, it is the result of sheer exhaustion, illness, or depression. Psychologist Stephanie Simonton has suggested that illness is the only acceptable form of meditation in America. Our bodies and minds have their ways of insisting. Is it possible that current epidemic levels of chronic fatigue and depression might be symptomatic of our collective need for rest? Could it be that symptoms that force us to slow, rest, sleep, or dream have an important, underlying healing function?

Depression, often referred to as the common cold of mental illness, remains at epidemic levels in industrialized nations around the world. Unlike the common cold, however, its symptoms can be protracted and debilitating. Despite the fact that most forms of depression have cyclical features—sometimes prominent and sometimes more subtle—there is little attention paid to the role of dysrhythmias in understanding and treating depression. Instead, the most popular interventions today are SSRIs (selective serotonin reuptake inhibitors), a class of stimulating drugs dubiously labeled "antidepressants."

On the surface, it might appear reasonable to treat depression with stimulating medications. But this approach disregards the larger social, psychological, and even spiritual picture of this condition. Buddhist philosophy teaches that depression results from excessive activation that is not properly balanced by rest. In our terms, it is about broken BRAC. More than a century ago, a handful of radical physicians were treating what we would call depression with an intervention called the *rest cure*. Although this controversial prescription for overly stringent bed rest received mixed reviews, it echoes a philosophical notion that we may want to reconsider today.

Whatever else symptoms of depression might indicate, they reflect the psyche's insistence that we rest. We might think of depression as psychology's answer to a fever, a reflection of the psyche's intent to self-heal. If we do not suppress its symptoms with stimulant medications, the fatigue that so commonly accompanies depression asks that we excuse ourselves from the world of activity, turn inward, and rest. I have come to believe that beyond all of the complex clinical features associated with it, being depressed is also a spiritual call for deep rest. Allowing ourselves to honor the call to rest not only supports healthier sleep but also opens a mysterious portal to the rich inner world of dreams, including the waking dream. If, as classic psychodynamic theory has long be-lieved, depression is about the loss of our dreams, rest is a sensible treatment.

The denial of our incessant drive and dysrhythmias are key symp-toms of our night blindness. Carl Jung taught that "awareness is healing." Expanding our awareness of the role of rhythms in our daily lives will help us heal our nights and night conscious-ness. With greater awareness, come greater options. Unlike pen-dulum clocks, we are not at the mercy of larger more dominant clocks/zeitgebers in the vicinity. We can consciously disengage from dysrhythmic aspects of culture and entrain to more health-supporting features of nature. We can consciously choose the trains we board, the kinds of rhythms we open ourselves to, and what we will resonate with in our lives. We can choose to rein-state rest into our lives.

Rhythm and Rest Practices

The following exercises are offered to help you become more sen-sitive to rest, rhythm, and resonance in your daily life. Developing such sensitivity is an essential foundation for healing one's night consciousness.

The Rest of Your Life

Practice simply being more aware of your inner reactions—both thoughts and feelings—to your need for rest. Are you even aware of these sensations? Try to specifically identify the sensations you experience as a call for rest. How does fatigue feel in your body? How does it affect your mind? Do you routinely regard such sen-sations or dismiss them? What kinds of thoughts might you have about others when they rest? Consider making notes about your observations and insights related to rest for a period of two to three weeks, preferably during a routine period of your life.

Monitor Your Pace

If you were a car, what kind of car would you be? Would you be sporty, a sedan, maybe an SUV? What is your top speed? And how are your brakes?

Practice becoming more conscious of your general tempo or pace—the timing in your life. Whatever it is you are doing, be aware of the manner in which you do it. This can be achieved by noting the adverbs that inform your actions. For example, might you be moving quickly, thinking slowly, acting considerately, or proceeding mindlessly? Think about the specific adverbs you associate with the kind of car you would be. Consider maintaining a journal of your observations and insights about the pace or timing of your life.

Become Mindful of Entrainment

Give some consideration to what you are resonating with and entrained to in your life. In addition to your circadian wake and sleep pattern, think about the basic energetic tempo of people you affiliate with and how that affects the tempo of your life.

Pay attention to the infradian rhythms that influence your daily life. These would include things like the music you listen to, the hobbies you engage in, and the athletic activities you are interested in. All of these have unique rhythmic signatures that can influence the quality of your life. These are the trains you ride. Are they bullet trains or slow trains? Give some thought to whether they are taking you where you really want to go. Are you enjoying the ride?

Take Time Out of Mind

Practice becoming extemporal. In other words, play with stepping out of your ordinary sense of time. Take part of a day, a full day, or even a long weekend to experiment with resynchronizing with your inner clock. Take your watch off and cover your clocks to avoid any temptation. Allow yourself to do what you want when you are inclined to. Be active, rest, eat, sleep, meditate, or do absolutely nothing as you wish. You might consider experimenting with keeping your watch off for some time even after you complete this experiment.

Notice Your Breath

Without trying to change or alter it in any way, practice simply becoming aware of your breathing throughout the day. Become aware of the rhythm as well as the depth of your breathing. The breath is an exceptional gauge of our personal timing, the momentary rhythmic process that determines our pace or tempo. You might allow your attention to shift to your breath when you find yourself tempted to check the time. Think of this as checking your personal sense of *timing*.

~

There are few spiritual school zones left in modern life. There are few places where we must legally slow down, where rest is enforced. When we do, we become more open and receptive to our deeper nature. Ecclesiastes is about remembering the essence of myth, the process of recurrence, of restoration, of life's essential rhythmicity. It is about conscious resonance with another world, a world beyond the intrusive pounding and screeching of industrial demands. A new and more conscious regard for rhythm, resonance, and rest is our ticket on another train—one with a sleeping car.

~3

Dusk: Surrendering to Sleep

Why is it that night falls, but then day breaks?
—GEORGE CARLIN

ONE SEPTEMBER EVENING several years ago I returned home from work to find that my electricity was out. A notice at my front door advised me that my bill was unpaid and my power had been turned off. Using my cell phone, I determined that there had been a glitch in the automatic payment deduction from my checking account, and I was told, after a considerable delay, it would not be possible to reinstate my power until the following day. I shrugged, lit a few candles, and realizing I could not listen to the evening news, reflexively went to turn on my desktop computer. Then it struck me—I felt robbed.

The consequences of having no electricity hit me one bit at a time. Like a burglary victim, I kept discovering new, unanticipated losses. I was unable to use my computer or watch television. I could not listen to music. The food in my refrigerator was starting to go bad, and I could not cook. I was not able talk on my landline. And because of the long conversation with the power company, my cell phone battery was drained, and I was unable to charge it. Within a short time, the backup battery for my security system also went out.

Despite the candlelight, it was getting hard to see anything in the house clearly. And with all of these little losses also went a certain sense of my personal power, my social connectedness, and the basic security I had taken for granted. I felt surprisingly powerless, frustrated, and quite lost.

I collapsed on the couch to consider my options.

The wide-scale power outages of the northeastern United States that left millions without electricity came to mind. I tried to imagine how people had handled those dilemmas. Then I recalled a report about the remarkable surge of births that occurred exactly nine months later. Hmm. But I was alone.

It was surprisingly disconcerting to meet the evening head on like this. Without power and light I had no way of buffering the dark and quiet. I felt disoriented and somewhat immobilized. My struggle was not just with the darkness but also with an eerie sense that there was no energy sizzling within my walls. I became aware of a previously unnoticed association between energy streaming into and through my home and my personal sense of power.

Although this felt a bit threatening at first, in just a few moments it was as if my vision, like my eyesight, began to adjust to the darkness. Looking around, I saw my home in a different light, literally. I realized that I simply was not accustomed to being in such a dark space with my eyes open. Few if any of my possessions called to me. Gone was the usual beckoning of an unfinished magazine article on the coffee table, the unopened mail, a thirsty plant, the telephone, the computer. My living room had filled with large, fuzzy shadows—everything in the outer world was rounded, softened, and, actually, not that interesting.

Without all of the common evening distractions, my attention was naturally drawn inward. I noticed that my breath had slowed and deepened. As my initial anxieties continued to diminish, the darkness had a deeply quieting effect. It occurred to me for the first time that darkness was more than the absence of light. I began appreciating an odd, palpable sense of stillness. Darkness was kind, spacious, and inviting. It was rest made visible.

But, really—I had more important things to do. A few moments later I found myself sitting up in bed with my laptop, two battery-operated camping lanterns flanking me, and a portable radio crackling nightly news at my feet. I could not help noticing how very dependent I was on electricity and artificial light, and even more so on the incessant stimulation and activity they encouraged.

Still, it started me wondering about deeply held cultural and personal policies regarding night and light. I remembered my mother's "What's the best thing in the world?" game and her sweet welcoming posture toward dusk and night. I began to realize how uncomfortable it was to meet the night on its own terms. And, despite my initial anxiety, I later drifted into an unusually deep and refreshing night's sleep.

In the coming weeks I began experimenting with a recommendation that I previously had offered only to my insomnia patients. An hour or so before bed, I significantly dimmed the lights all around my home. I began to simulate dusk. And I was surprised to discover the deeply transformative power inherent in this simple practice.

Reconsidering Dusk

Dusk is disorienting. It is that sudden, anticipatory hush that settles upon an audience when the house lights start to dim. Drawing our attention from the scattered din of active daytime concerns, dusk invites us inward to the focused, quiet performance of night. If we are willing, dusk will gently reorient us from our ordinary daytime consciousness to a nonordinary night consciousness.

Falling asleep is a gradual process that begins long before bedtime. An honest encounter with dusk teaches us that it is the environmental analogue of sleep onset. By nature, we go down gradually with the sun. Although it has been the preoccupation of much sleep research, trying to define the onset of sleep is like trying to define the onset of night. In nature night does not fall, it only slowly descends. Despite appearances, neither do we simply "fall" asleep.

Reflecting the common belief that sleep onset occurs with the flick of a switch, sleep science has established conventions that try to pinpoint the exact moment we fall asleep. Studies that seek to confirm a strictly objective definition of sleep onset, however, fail to find strong correlations with subjective reports of sleep or wakefulness. Although much of our scientific understanding and medical management of sleep is based on being able to define when sleep begins and ends, we need to keep in mind that these definitions are somewhat arbitrary.

When we open to dusk, we learn that natural sleep does not occur in a flash. There is no "night fall." Sleep, like night, descends only gradually, gently surrendering the day. Likewise, from an EEG perspective, the transition from waking beta states to the deep Stage 3 and 4 sleep of theta and delta states carries us through a darkening dreamlike passageway—a personal twilight zone. Referred to as *hypnagogia,* which suggests a movement toward sleep, this transition involves a fundamental dissolution of waking consciousness, of our ordinary sense of self. Just as day is dissolving into night, our waking consciousness, or ego, is also dissolving into our deeper self.

Whisking us through a narrow channel of dream imagery, this dissolution is the alchemical gateway to sleeping consciousness. Unlike the more cohesive dreams that will visit later in the night, these hypnagogic sleep onset dreams are typically brief, bizarre, and unsettling. They usually include a kaleidoscopic sequence of rapidly morphing images, emerging and dissolving. They do, indeed, unsettle our waking hold on the world. Interestingly, though we all normally move through a sleep-onset dream experience nightly, most people retain little if any conscious memory of such experiences.

The hypnagogic dream may be accompanied by sleep starts associated with a sense of falling and reflecting the ego's experience of letting go. Most of us do not proceed consciously through our personal twilight zone. Directly witnessing the dissolution of our waking selves would leave many of us queasy.

Informed by a mechanistic view of life, our contemporary take on sleep onset is that it is a lights out or a sudden dead-to-the-world phenomenon. We expect sleep to come on our terms, at the flick of a switch. As if we were cars, we want to just hit the brakes when we please, stop, and turn the engine off. We declare ourselves great sleepers when we can *go out like a light* the moment our head hits the pillow.

Unfortunately, far too many of us do not apply the brakes until we are already in the garage; we fail to slow sufficiently before getting into bed. The more natural, slow and easy transition through dusk has been replaced by a crashing approach to sleep. Some people just roll along until they run out of gas, and others simply knock themselves out with the help of chemical emergency brakes, including sedating substances like alcohol and sleeping pills.

Such a common mechanistic posture toward the hypnagogic transition inevitably fails us, leaving tens of millions of people silently struggling to fall asleep night after night. Our mechanistic posture ignores the critical and meaningful subjective, personal, and essentially mythic aspects of night and sleep onset. We need to reconsider the mythic dimensions of night and sleep. We need a rapprochement with Nyx.

Born of the primordial void, Chaos, the Greek goddess Nyx wielded immense power, even among gods. In the Orphic Creation myth, she ruled with her father, Protogonus, who appointed her as the supreme ruler of heaven and earth. According to Homer's *Iliad*, Nyx was the only goddess that Zeus truly feared. Not surprisingly, Nyx was nocturnal, dwelling in the Underworld by day and emerging at dusk to unveil night. In a black, star-studded gown, she traversed the sky, darkening and cooling the planet in preparation for slumber. And at her side was her son, Hypnos, the god of sleep.

In modern times the mythic forces of Nyx and Hypnos, the spiritual embodiments of night and sleep, have been transposed and reduced to the scientific machinations of neurochemistry. Most of us are now familiar with melatonin, the neurohormone that mediates night, sleep, and dreams. Melatonin is a primordial molecule, having evolved very early in the emergence of life on Earth. Released when Descartes' "third-eye," the pineal gland, "sees" that it is getting dark out, melatonin is essentially nocturnal. It also plays a powerful role in managing our biology, informing the body and brain of the arrival and presence of night. Much like Nyx ascending into the night sky, melatonin levels rise through the night, cooling our bodies and inviting sleep and dreams. Like Nyx, melatonin is primordial, powerful, nocturnal, and soporific. And, as we will see, like Nyx, melatonin has been severely suppressed.

As important as our scientific understanding of sleep is, attempting to reduce what is clearly mythic to what is merely mechanistic diminishes the immensity of night and obscures sleep's true nature, personal meaning, and spirit.

Night Light and Night Life

Excessive light at night (LAN) is psychologically and spiritually blinding. As in a theater, it is difficult to clearly see the activity on stage when the house lights are on. Most of us are, however, habituated to and deeply dependent on such light. LAN may not have the obviously stimulating effect of a cup of coffee after dinner, but therein lies its danger. It is subtle and pernicious. Because it significantly impedes our experience of dusky consciousness, I believe that excessive LAN may be the most critical, overlooked factor in sleep onset problems.

LAN interferes with the natural process of sleep onset by both energizing us and inhibiting the release of melatonin. Light can energize us by boosting brain levels of serotonin, a neurochemical that regulates mood and energy. Even relatively small amounts of light at night can hamper the release of melatonin, delay our sleep phase, and interfere with our slowing and sleep onset. Although we may be aware that it is night, when melatonin release is delayed or inhibited, our biology does not get the message, leaving our brains and bodies functioning as if it is still daytime. Beyond energizing us and inhibiting melatonin, LAN literally lights the way for us to engage in a wide range of sleep-inhibiting activities at night.

Millions of Americans are overactive, overeat, overdrink, and watch too much television at night. Night life is commonly characterized by the extensive use of mood-altering substances, excessive food consumption, and distracting and dramatic entertainment. Frequently, it involves an incessant and unwieldy mental pace—the bop-until-you-drop approach to evening. In these ways, prime time distracts us, preventing our natural surrender to dusk, night, and our personal shadows. It incites us by cranking up the volume of our energies just when we need quiet. And all this noise impedes our slowing and sleep onset.

According to the National Sleep Foundation (2004), 90 percent of Americans watch television or listen to the radio one hour before going to bed. Over 40 percent of adults polled stated that they often delay their bedtime to watch television or surf the Web. Sixty-three percent of us report reading in the last hour before bed. And 15 percent of adults report exercising in the last hour before going to bed, despite common knowledge that exercise raises core body temperature, which interferes with sleep onset.

As I stated previously, evening appears to be the most common period of substance use. For many, given work schedules and social demands, it is their only opportunity. Evening substance use is generally about applying *chemical brakes* to help slow the bullet train of our waking lives and to buffer our encounter with darkness. The most common substances used at night are alcohol, marijuana, and, of course, sleeping pills. And for those of us averse to using substances, overeating can do the trick.

More than 90 percent of Americans use alcohol in one form or another—mostly at night. Although the initial effect of alcohol consumption is mild stimulation, it is a central nervous system depressant that will eventually slow us down. For many, alcohol is dusk in a bottle—a chemical backup braking system. Many people believe that alcohol actually helps them sleep. Although it may appear to facilitate sleep onset, alcohol suppresses melatonin, alters our circadian rhythms, and significantly disrupts sleep and dreaming later in the night.

Alcohol abuse and dependence are associated with chronic disruptions of sleep and dreaming. Kirk J. Brower, a psychiatrist at the University of Michigan Alcohol Research Center and executive director of the Chelsea Arbor Treatment Center in Ann Arbor, summarizes his findings of a comprehensive review of research on sleep and alcoholism for the National Institute on Alcohol Abuse and Alcoholism:

> Sleep problems, which can have significant clinical and economic consequences, are more common among alcoholics than among nonalcoholics. During both drinking periods and withdrawal, alcoholics commonly experience problems falling asleep and decreased total sleep time. . . . Even alcoholics who have been abstinent for short periods of time (i.e., several weeks) or extended periods of time (i.e., several years) may experience persistent sleep abnormalities. Researchers also found that alcoholics are more likely to suffer from certain sleep disorders, such as sleep apnea. Conversely, sleep problems may predispose some people to developing alcohol problems. Furthermore, sleep problems may increase the risk of relapse among abstinent alcoholics. (2001, 1)

I believe that people active in alcohol recovery programs could benefit from a firm commitment to improve the quality of their nights, sleep, and dreaming. Interestingly, many of the psychological and spiritual principles and practices that support healthy sleep and dreaming are, in fact, consistent with those found in 12-step and related recovery programs.

Over the past thirty years, marijuana has become a popular, albeit illegal, alternative chemical braking system. Although less is known about the impact of marijuana on sleep onset than is known about alcohol, marijuana users commonly report that it helps them slow down, relax, and prepare for sleep. A number of surveys reveal that millions of Americans, particularly teenagers and young adults, use marijuana on a daily basis. Some studies suggest that, like alcohol, marijuana may in fact promote sleep onset but later compromise the quality of sleep. However, given that marijuana dramatically increases our endogenous melatonin, it is not a surprise that other studies contradict these findings and suggest that this substance actually promotes sleep. While uncertainty remains about its effect on sleep, marijuana use is associated with increased appetite. Research has confirmed that it lowers blood sugar, increasing food cravings and, potentially, excessive nighttime eating.

But we certainly do not need to smoke marijuana to eat excessively at night. Many people routinely have their largest meals in the evening. And we do not stop there. We continue to nibble, munch, and snack right up until bedtime. The National Sleep Foundation (2004) reports that 43 percent of Americans eat something in the last hour before bed. Eating triggers a parasympathetic or relaxation response in our nervous system that helps us slow down. Excessive late eating, however, backfires by disrupting our circadian cycles. Since it is out of sync with our digestive system's expectations, it confuses our personal clock and predisposes us to gastroesophageal reflux, a sleep-disruptive digestive disorder, which we will discuss later.

The National Sleep Foundation (2004) also reports that 21 percent of U.S. adults drink caffeinated beverages at night, including cola drinks, teas, and coffee. Caffeine energizes us and simultaneously inhibits the action of adenosine, one of the brain's secondary sleep-inducing neurochemicals. Because caffeine has a long "half-life," its sleep-inhibiting effects can extend up to ten or more hours, depending on the amount and timing of its consumption.

These kinds of night life activities impair our relationship with dusk and can damage our sleep phase. LAN functions to hold back night until we deem sleep admissible, at which point, with the extinction of the last light on our bed stand, we expect night to fall. We expect sleep to arrive, promptly on cue, when we are good and ready. Millions of us do manage to crash from the sheer exhaustion associated with life at chronic warp speed. But by ignoring the gentle, soporific promptings of dusk, millions of us must rely on substances and food to artificially induce sleep. Although we remain largely unaware of it, the quality of sleep we obtain in this way is seriously compromised.

Going to Sleep Sideways

When my granddaughter Claire was four, she stayed late at my home one night while her parents attended a concert. We sat on the sofa watching her favorite cartoons right through her bedtime. Despite being obviously sleepy, she insisted that she was not yet ready for bed. Children seem to learn very early on that there is some distinct value in staying up late. I suppose it is because they observe adults routinely do so.

Sleepy-eyed, Claire finally turned to me and said, "Papa, I'm just gonna rest my head like this on your lap, OK? I'm not gonna sleep."

"That's OK, sweetie," I said.

A few seconds later she lifted her heavy head and looked up at me through big, bleary eyes to say, "I'm still awake, Papa. I'm just gonna close my eyes to rest them just a little bit. I'm not gonna sleep, OK?"

"That's fine, sweetie," I said. "Would you like me to leave the TV on? . . . Claire?"

She was out.

My observations suggest that adults who are reluctant or unable to consciously let go of waking routinely rely on similar sleep onset strategies. With the aid of a book, television, the radio, or other bedtime activities that distract us from directly surrendering to our sleepiness, we simply trick ourselves to sleep. We approach sleep sideways, intentionally resisting it as it arises until it builds sufficient momentum to just push us over the edge. When the lights finally go out, others engage in classic mind games like counting sheep or doing math problems until their sleep momentum reaches its necessary threshold. It is like a spring-loaded mechanism designed to instantaneously catapult us over our personal twilight zones directly into sleep.

Why do we do this? I believe that *most people are reluctant to spend a few moments alone with themselves*—in the dark. As I suggested earlier, people frequently declare themselves good sleepers when they *go out like a light* the moment their head hits the pillow.

Falling asleep in a flash, however, is not a sign of being a good sleeper; it is a sign that one is carrying an excessive sleep debt. In fact, if persistent, it is likely a symptom of a sleep disorder.

Taking twenty or thirty minutes to gradually slip into sleep after the lights go out is perfectly natural and healthy. Unconsciously maintaining an excessive sleep debt, however, may have a protective function. It ushers us instantaneously through hypnagogia, through our personal twilight zones. It allows us to circumvent underlying anxieties that emerge opportunistically as we drift into sleep.

I believe that over time most people habituate to such avoidant strategies. Eventually, their braking system will wear down, and the struggle to fall asleep will intensify. The sleep onset anxieties held back by our bedtime activities will eventually rebound as insomnia.

During any given night on this planet, tens of millions of people struggle with falling asleep. According to the National Sleep Foundation (2005), at least one in five American adults routinely has trouble falling asleep at least a few nights a week. They watch the clock as minutes churn slowly into hours. They worry, ache, toss, turn, count sheep, pray, get up, get down, walk around, move to another room, give up, work on their computers, eat leftovers, drink milk, take a drink, and take sleeping pills.

Taking Something to Sleep

Michael arrived in my office with chronic, intractable sleep onset insomnia. As a physician's assistant, he had ready access to sleeping medications as well as knowledge about alternative sleep aids. He admitted to tinkering with a range of prescription, over-the-counter, and alternative sleep aids for more than a decade. Most of what he tried seemed to work for a while, but then his sleep would inevitably deteriorate again. Michael succeeded in gradually weaning himself from dependence on a prescription sleeping pill he was taking at the time. But despite the fact that his sleep subsequently improved with psychological and behavioral changes, he slipped back into the habit of taking sleep aids. "I don't know why," he confessed in one of our sessions. "I just feel like I need to take something to sleep." Michael, like many people I have worked with, had developed dependence not only on specific sleeping pills but also on the belief that he needed to *take something to sleep*.

The most common medical treatment offered to people with insomnia is sleeping pills. The idea of *taking something to sleep* is ancient. Hypnos is often depicted in deep repose in the mouth of a cave on the shore of the Aegean Sea—surrounded by beds of wild red poppies. A wide range of botanicals have been used to induce sleep in virtually all cultures around the world since the start of time. Modern medicine puts a scientific spin on this tradition, designing sleeping pills, or *hypnotics* (after Hypnos), that tamper with our neurological waking or braking systems in complex and often poorly understood ways. Unfortunately, most sleeping pills offer only a temporary fix that simply conceals underlying symptoms. And then they backfire.

Despite the obvious fact that sleep onset is a gradual process, given their adherence to the mechanistic view, sleep scientists keep looking for that elusive sleep onset mechanism. Because we are machines, the belief seems to be, there must be a switch somewhere. There must be a biological button or a neurochemical knob that would allow us to control the sleep-wake process. It would allow us to turn off waking and turn on sleep the way we do lights or cars or computers. If we could locate this switch, the belief goes, we could wipe out insomnia.

It is questionable, however, if what we get from a sleeping pill is really sleep. For the most part, both prescription and over-the-counter sleeping pills do not result in natural sleep—they offer an artificial or *simulated sleep*. Most of them actually inhibit deeper stages of sleep, constrict dreaming, and result in dependence, if not outright addiction. After discontinuation, sleeping pill users frequently experience serious *rebound insomnias*, leaving them in worse shape than before they began taking the pills. Most sleeping pills are not much more than chemical knockout agents. And sleeping pills are particularly hard on us as we age. Often their effects linger throughout the morning and even into the day, compromising our cognitive abilities and our very consciousness.

Perhaps most alarming is evidence suggesting that chronic sleeping pill use is associated with increased mortality. Sleep specialist Daniel Kripke, at the University of California, San Diego, addresses this crucial topic in his book *The Dark Side of Sleeping Pills*. Committed to exposing the serious dangers of these medications, he has made his book available free of charge at his Web site (see bibliography). Dr. Kripke reviews research supporting his belief that the chronic use of sleep medication is linked to significant increases in mortality.

Despite all of these concerns, growing numbers of Americans continue to use sleeping pills. The National Sleep Foundation (2005) found that 15 percent of Americans reported using prescription and/or over-the-counter sleep medications at least a few nights each week. Their data also indicate that sleeping pill use has continued to rise steadily in recent years.

Virtually all sleep doctors agree that sleeping pills are meant only for short-term use and should be administered as part of a larger, comprehensive sleep health program. Given the tremendous shortage of sleep doctors, however, this is rarely achieved in practice. So, why do we continue to use them? There are two reasons.

First, they are a source of tremendous revenue for the pharmaceutical industry. Sleeping pills and related sedatives represent a significant and steadily growing market around the world. A number of newer sleeping pills are now under development, promising more sophisticated chemical knockouts and even greater profits. Drug companies have launched extensive media campaigns to convince both doctors and the public that such medications are safe and appropriate. Some estimates suggest that sleeping pill sales will triple over the next five years.

Second, we use sleeping pills because they meet our very naive criterion for defining sleep. They knock us out.

In the end, beyond whatever damage these drugs may be doing

to our bodies, they also harm us psychologically and spiritually. When used as a primary treatment for chronic sleeplessness, sleeping pills inevitably undermine our self-efficacy—our own ability to allow sleep to come naturally. Taking pills to switch on sleep reinforces the notion that we are machines and distracts us from a deeper understanding of the sacred process of sleep onset.

For those occasions when a short-term sleep aid is indicated, a number of alternative, over-the-counter sleep-promoting substances are available that appear to be effective and less harmful than standard sleeping pills. Some of these, like valerian, are time-honored remedies that have been used for centuries, while others, like 5-HTP and tryptophan, are more recent scientific discoveries. Sometimes referred to as natural sleep aids, these substances have generally been shown to support more natural sleep patterns, have fewer side effects, and work in greater tandem with our natural rhythms.

Letting Go of Something to Sleep

I believe that most sleep onset difficulties stem from our reluctance to rest—to slow down, encounter dusk, and let go of the day's emotional residue before getting into bed. Failing to do so builds a backlog of unprocessed emotions and anxiety that threatens to emerge when we slow sufficiently to try to sleep.

Usually unaware of what is really impeding their sleep, many people spiral into a vicious cycle of confusion and anxiety. The more they cannot sleep, the more they worry. And the more they worry, the more they cannot sleep. But the fact that millions of people become anxious about falling asleep at night too easily obscures the fact that they were probably anxious to begin with. I believe that sleep onset difficulties can be best understood in terms of suppressed anxiety.

A common symptom of sleep onset anxiety is an involuntary pattern of intrusive and incessant thinking that I call *cognitive popcorn*. After a moment of quiet in bed, thoughts begin to pop spontaneously into awareness. Like popcorn popping on the stove top, these thoughts quickly multiply. Most often they appear to be relatively mundane and benign, about various and sundry things, and certainly not warranting their co-opting precious sleep time. The body wants to sleep, but the mind's engine keeps going and going, producing background noise that inhibits sleep onset.

Deborah was a handsome and strong woman in her early sixties who had been struggling with sleep onset problems for more than four years. She explained that she had "read all the books" and was "doing everything right" but was still consistently taking hours to fall asleep. As a routine part of my evaluation of her insomnia, I asked about possible precipitating factors, about what was happening in her life around the time her problem began. She thought for a moment. "Well, it was a difficult period," she said. "My husband had been in an accident and required so much of my attention. But that was four years ago," she quickly added. "It's not something I even think about anymore."

"What goes on inside your head when you're trying to sleep, then?" I asked.

"Nothing . . . nothing, really," she replied.

"Your mind is just blank?" I asked.

"Well, no . . . no, actually, I just start to think about different things. You know, nothing important. Last night I remember thinking about needing to get the oil changed in the car and things like that. I don't know why I think about all this silly stuff," she said with frustration. "But I can't seem to stop it."

"When you say you think about all this, do you actually intentionally choose to think these thoughts?" I asked.

"No. Of course not. It's strange. They just pop into my head. I don't know why. It makes no sense at all."

As we continued, I asked if her sleep difficulties ever affected her husband's sleep. Deborah grew visibly anxious and choked on her words to hold back tears. "My husband died three years ago." She began to weep softly. "From injuries related to his accident," she added. "Gosh, I'm just surprised to be crying. I . . . I thought all this was behind me for some time now." She dropped her head and cried for another moment or two before regaining her composure.

Early the next morning I received a message from Deborah on my voice mail. "I think we opened Pandora's box," she said. "I ended up crying myself to sleep. But, frankly," she continued, "it was the best night's sleep I've had in a long time. And I just can't figure out why."

I believe cognitive popcorn is symptomatic of deferred and deflected anxiety. Whether deeply held shadow issues, concerns that accrue in the course of daily life, or unexamined grief, as was the case with Deborah, when emotions are not adequately processed, they become a source of psychological heat. Like the flame beneath a kettle of popcorn, this underlying heat may not be visible, but it is persistently popping cognitions into our awareness. Turning down the heat—identifying and releasing the underlying emotion—can be of significant benefit. Uncomfortable as it might be, crying oneself to sleep is one way to get there. I will recommend a basic strategy for addressing cognitive popcorn in the practices section at the close of this chapter.

Although I believe anxiety, manifesting as cognitive popcorn, is the most common factor contributing to sleep onset insomnia, I do not mean to oversimplify the causes of this condition. Insomnias are complex and may be associated with a variety of other biological factors as well. Many people struggle with digestive problems, chronic pain, and allergic reactions. Many others struggle with *restless leg syndrome* (RLS), a debilitating condition that interferes with sleep onset by causing uncomfortable sensations in one's legs when attempting to rest. Previously, we saw that when our personal clock runs slower than outer clocks, we may experience a delayed sleep phase disorder, trying in vain to fall asleep during subjective waking time. To varying degrees, these conditions may also represent an indirect, opportunistic biological emergence of suppressed daytime anxieties. In any event, they generally require professional attention.

Night as Sleep Medicine

An open and honest encounter with dusk offers a much-needed alternative to prime time and the knockout approach to sleep. If we reinstate it into our lives, dusk will naturally encourage us to slow down and rest. In signaling the end of daylight and the start of night, dusk provides a resounding beat in the rhythm of the day. It calls for a shift in consciousness and behavior that helps us negotiate darkness and night. Dusk offers gracious assistance, if we resonate with it, in our nightly need to let go of waking and surrender to sleep. Dusk calls for a new kind of nightmindedness—for personal ritual and expanded spiritual awareness to promote greater lucidity.

A more healthful and spiritually sensitive approach to dusk and sleep onset involves three steps. First, we must intentionally deluminate, that is, dim our lights at night to slow down. Second, we must be prepared, through the use of evening ritual, to embrace and heal anxieties that naturally emerge when we slow. And, third, we must learn how to surrender to sleep.

Delumination

Night is a sight for sore eyes. It offers our vision a rest. Dusk begins to turn down the volume of the visual world, which often gets cranked up without our even noticing. Most relaxation techniques call upon us to eliminate or at least reduce external visual stimulation by closing our eyes. But could it be that we might actually need a certain amount of exposure to darkness with our eyes open? Is it possible that we actually have a darkness deficiency? Recent research suggests that exposure to darkness is important in modulating our circadian rhythms. Other studies of visual sensory deprivation show promise in promoting general healing. Most compelling, however, are findings from an extensive study of the history of sleep patterns.

In his book *At Day's Close: Night in Times Past* (2005), historian A. Roger Ekirch examines the night lives of people who lived between two hundred and five hundred years ago, long before the use of excessive artificial lighting. He discovered that Europeans of this era routinely spent significantly more time awake and active in dim and dark spaces than we do today. Additional research along these lines by Thomas Wehr (1999) of the National Institute of Mental Health suggests there may be significant health and mental health benefits associated with this kind of exposure to darkness. (We will discuss Ekirch's and Wehr's work in more detail as we proceed.)

When I keep my lights dim in the evening, I instinctively move more slowly. I find myself speaking more slowly and softly, and my thought processes seem to slow as well. It is simply unsafe to move quickly through dim or dark spaces. Psychologists have long known that an intentional slowing of external behavior is usually followed by comparable slowing of internal experience.

Dusk also encourages community—a kind of social huddling. People universally come together at night for safety and support. With the distractions of the outside world fading, dusk offers a kind of intimacy less accessible by day. Diminished LAN means less reading, television, and other activities that can be socially isolating. We can focus on one another more easily at dusk and in the evening. Whether as friends, as families, or in a romantic way, as lovers, dusk encourages us to connect more deeply and directly with one another than we are typically capable of doing by the light of day.

Evening Ritual and Prayer

Dusk can be unsettling. Given both its psychological challenges and sacred possibilities, it is not surprising that spiritual and religious traditions from around the world have evolved evening rituals that provide support and guidance through the transition into night and sleep.

By evening ritual, I am referring to a range of practices that encourage a conscious rapprochement with dusk and night. These can include traditional prayer and spiritual practices as well as psychological or personal approaches such as cleansing and relaxation techniques. Evening ritual is about creating a structure, not a substitution, for a personal encounter with dusk. To be effective, it needs to be regular and rhythmic. As we saw previously, rhythm is comforting; it helps us feel safe. Ritual is the behavioral expression of rhythmicity.

Prayer is probably the most universal and common evening and bedtime ritual. Every major religious and spiritual tradition provides special nightly prayers that acknowledge both the challenge and potential of letting go of waking and opening to sleep. In *Entering the Temple of Dreams,* Tamar Frankiel and Judy Greenfeld consider this notion from a Jewish perspective:

> [T]he most profound and powerful aspect of the change (from waking to sleeping) is that we must abandon conscious control of our lives. . . . This can generate great anxiety and is particularly threatening to the ego. . . . There is a letting go or suspending of ego, which scans, patrols, protects us from life's dangers. Our sages recommended the Bedtime Prayers as a cloak of protection and reassurance for the body and the ego. (2000, 21–22)

Evening ritual and prayer provide an essential structure to help us negotiate the challenges of dusk and darkness. They help carry us across the sacred threshold from waking toward sleep, but they do not actually deliver us to sleep. Evening ritual and prayer simply help us invoke sleep.

Letting Go of Waking

People generally approach sleep like it is a volitional act, as if they can simply choose to go there. "I'm going to sleep" is a common expression. It suggests that the state of sleep exists in some location that one can intentionally access at will. Anyone who has experienced even just one night of insomnia has been instantly disabused of this notion. We cannot "go to sleep." Sleep is not a place that we can intentionally access. We can go to the movies, to the bathroom, or to work. We can go to bed. But we cannot literally go to sleep. This kind of volitional thinking is misleading, and because it activates the mind, it can actually backfire and impede the onset of sleep.

Sleep onset is not an act of volition. All of our preparation for sleep, including evening ritual and prayer, is like ordering a pizza. We take the necessary action—we make the call, place the order, and prepare for its arrival. And then we wait. We do not go out in search of the delivery guy. If we do, we are liable to miss him. Keeping an eye out for the sandman—actively pursuing sleep onset—will interfere with its arrival. I believe the simplest yet the most difficult aspect of getting to sleep is the surrender of one's volition.

When we speak of "falling asleep," then, we may be closer to the truth. In letting go of waking, we drop and fall into the state of sleep. For most of us, however, waking is the gold standard for consciousness, for existence, for being alive. Intentionally letting go of waking—surrendering our very sense of being—is a fundamentally frightening notion. In letting go of waking, we let go of our ordinary sense of self and, metaphorically, we die. Don Quixote speaks of this uncomfortable association: "Now blessings light on him that first invented this same sleep. . . . There is only one thing, which somebody once put into my head, that I dislike in sleep; it is that it resembles death; there is very little difference between a man in his first sleep, and a man in his last sleep."

The association of falling asleep and dying is archetypal. Thanatos, the Greek god of death, was Hypnos's twin brother. Likewise, in Tibetan Buddhist philosophy the passage into sleep and into death are considered functionally synonymous. In his book *Sleeping, Dreaming, and Dying* (Varela 1997), the Dalai Lama emphasizes that the process of falling asleep closely approximates the psychological and spiritual experience of dying. This may explain why most of us fail to witness our own sleep onset process—that dreamlike hypnagogic state associated with the dissolution of the waking self.

It has been said that *nothing cures insomnia like the realization that it's time to get up.* Realizing that it is time to get up allows us to finally let go of our anxious desire to fall asleep. I believe it is this simple act of letting go that permits us to fall sleep. In the end, it does not matter how large or small a thing we let go of, only that we practice doing so nightly. All complexities aside, we come to understand that falling asleep is an act of faith.

Lucid Sleep Onset Practices

The following exercises are designed to help you experiment with and determine approaches to dusk and sleep onset that work best for you.

Open to Sleep

Overly stimulating evening activities, late and heavy eating, excessive alcohol consumption, and habitual use of sleeping pills all significantly compromise a natural sleep onset process. I recommend taking definite but gradual steps to manage or eliminate these problems from your night life.

Whatever evening activities you choose to engage in, be cognizant of the spirit with which they imbue your evening. Night is certainly not the best time to partake of the news, a murder mystery, monster movies, or industrial rock music.

Create a sacred space for sleep. Consider using feng shui, the ancient Eastern practice of organizing space for optimum well-being, to arrange your bedroom furnishings in a sleep-conducive manner. Light, heat, and noise are common sleep thieves. Make sure your sleeping area is dark, cool, and quiet throughout the night. It is important that the bedroom feel psychologically safe and "timeless." Do whatever you need to promote a sense of complete safety. This might mean installing a security system, obtaining a protective icon, hanging your grandmother's quilt over the headboard, or getting a dog. Never check the time when you are unable to sleep. Reposition any clocks in your bedroom to minimize the temptation.

In the end, whatever gets you through the night is worthy of your consideration. Short of obviously damaging behaviors, such as nightcaps or excessive illumination, consider personalizing your bed, bedroom, and sleep onset rituals. Some people find they feel more secure and sleep better with heavy bed covers. Even as adults, sleeping with stuffed animals is comforting for many. My father slept best near an open window, even through cold winters. Fortunately, my mother loved heavy covers.

Simulate Dusk

Dusk simulation refers to a set of key evening and sleep-onset promoting practices. I recommend that you personalize and gradually integrate dusk simulation practices into your lifestyle. Plan to experiment with dusk simulation for at least three or four consecutive nights at a time when it will not place undo pressure on anyone in your home.

Beginning about one hour before your bedtime, significantly dim or turn off most of the lights within and around your home, leaving only enough light for safety and basic maneuvering. If necessary, block out as much outdoor street light as you can. You may use candlelight or dimmed electric lighting, but only sparingly.

If other members of your household find it necessary to maintain normal levels of lighting, consider wearing dark, wraparound sunglasses as an alternative. This might seem strange, but you will likely adapt to it rather quickly. And in addition to reaping the spiritual and psychological benefits of dusk simulation, you will, of course, look pretty cool.

Sit down and take a few moments to adjust to your dusky surroundings, with your eyes open. Notice your mind's initial reaction to the darkening and shadows. Depending on personal history, people react to this experience in different ways. Some witness an internal dialogue that judges this activity as "a waste of time," "being silly," or "possibly dangerous." Others find it relaxing and enjoyable. Most people will likely experience a mix of both. Because dusk draws us deeply inward, it is not uncommon to become aware of childhood memories of evening—both positive and disturbing.

As you slow down and rest, let yourself become reacquainted with the natural advent of sleepiness. Just as light and darkness peacefully coexist in the form of dusk, sleepiness and wakefulness can peacefully coexist in our dusky consciousness. Spend some time experiencing this dusky consciousness. Notice the sensations throughout your body. What is happening with your muscles, your bones? How do your eyes feel? What kinds of thoughts and feelings arise? What is happening with your breath?

The mind commonly offers a running commentary on most of our experiences. Notice any judgments you might have about your diminishing energy. Let yourself honestly examine whatever feelings and judgments come. People often appraise their initial uneasiness with slowing down as boredom. Are you tempted to seek some kind of stimulation? Do you notice any unfinished business, entertainment options, or other distractions calling to you?

If reading is an evening activity you enjoy, consider using some type of attachable book light or a low-wattage bulb for illumination. Make sure the bulb is capped or covered, shielding your eyes from the light. If you choose to watch television or use a computer, experiment with dimming the brightness on your monitors. You will notice that television and computer monitors appear to emit relatively intense light when they are viewed in a darkened room.

When feasible, it is interesting and beneficial to experience dusk outdoors. This is virtually impossible to do if you are in a highly populated area where nights are automatically lit up and buzzing. If you are in a rural or a quiet residential area, however, there may be no need to simulate dusk. Merely allow nature to dim the light around you. When you are able, gaze at the night sky, allowing yourself to absorb its immense breadth.

Let Go of the Day

Dusk is an ideal time to gently process and let go of the day. We have all heard that our nighttime troubles will look much better in the light of day. Yet experienced in the context of a night that is welcomed rather than resisted, our daytime difficulties may actually look better in the shadowy light of dusk.

Whether alone with one's journal or together with loved ones, the softening influence and sense of containment offered by night can facilitate our processing of emotion. It is useful to begin by simply listing all the things you would like to let go of from the day.

How do you personally let go of something? Reframing it in the bigger picture? Practicing relaxation in the face of what you might be holding on to? Actively working on forgiving? Or just not giving something attention anymore? Meditations, visualizations, and other related practices designed to help in letting go are especially useful in the evening. I am particularly fond of Hugh Prather's compilation of "letting go" exercises in *The Little Book of Letting Go.*

Because we are not always able to let go of everything we would like to let go of at the end of the day, I have found it useful to let go even of the need to let go. Ultimately, it is less about what you let go of and more about the simple willingness to practice doing so. Make the last thing on your letting-go list letting go of the list itself.

Evening Ritual and Prayer

If we are open to it, evening ritual and prayer can help carry us graciously across that sacred bridge of evening to the threshold of sleep. I recommend that you experiment with and create personalized rituals that work for you. Include whatever traditional approaches you like, but add any quieting practices that feel meaningful and helpful.

Many people enjoy and benefit from evening cleansing rituals, warm baths, whirlpools, or showers. Changing out of daytime clothes associated with work or other activities into more comfortable nighttime garb can also be helpful. Many sacred traditions encourage evening meditation or contemplation. Still others recommend gentle forms of yoga to relax.

Storytelling may be the most common evening activity across cultures. It offers a way of debriefing or processing the day by re-framing it in the larger context of social meaning or cultural myth. Whether these are stories of personal experiences from earlier in the day or epic tales that have been handed across generations—or anything in-between—the healing benefits of storytelling are well established. Storytelling is found in diverse healing traditions ranging from shamanism to contemporary psychotherapies. Some experts believe that the process of storytelling is one of the major effective ingredients in 12-step recovery programs.

When it comes to bedtime prayer, many options are available from a wide range of spiritual and religious traditions. You can also personalize your prayer. For those who are open to it, bedtime prayers are helpful in addressing the sense of vulnerability associated with night and surrender to sleep. Whatever forms they may take, bedtime prayers usually remind us of a higher order, someone or something we feel safe letting go into. They help us conjure faith.

Manage Sleep-Related Anxiety

Cognitive popcorn is a common symptom of sleep onset anxieties and can be managed by a simple journaling exercise that encourages the release of underlying emotion. Begin by writing out a *thought sample.* Take a moment to jot brief notes about random thoughts traversing your mind. Your aim is to get a sampling of your thoughts, which, like a blood sample, is not meant to collect it all. Next, read what you have written, looking for any emotion embedded in these thoughts. Remember that cognitive popcorn results from the heat of these underlying emotions. You may notice sadness, anger, fear, or other feelings.

Once you have identified these feelings, sit with your eyes closed and allow whatever emotions you discover to simply wash over you. Surrender to them with no attempt at understanding, analyzing, judging, or changing them in any way. To do this, some people visualize themselves immersed in a whirlpool bath filled with their emotions in liquid form. Cognitive popcorn, fired by the heat of concealed emotions, will ease when this heat is released through acceptance of these emotions. This practice is most useful when done about thirty minutes before bed.

If you experience further difficulty in falling asleep, consider using the time-honored "4-7-8 breath," one of the most efficient ways of managing anxiety. Begin by placing the tip of your tongue against the ridge behind your upper front teeth. Slowly breathe in through your nose to the count of four. Hold your breath to the count of seven. Then breathe out through your mouth with a whooshing sound to the count of eight. Repeat this cycle four times, and then let go.

Surrender to Sleep

Think about the process of falling asleep as a personal spiritual practice—the practice of doing nothing, of surrendering volition and one's waking sense of self. There is nothing we have to do to sleep—except to let go of waking.

Practice lucid sleep onset by cultivating more awareness of the process of falling asleep, of your personal twilight zone. Remember that we are drawn through a brief hypnagogic dream during this transition. Casually observe the myriad of thoughts, feelings, images, bodily sensations, and other experiences as you surrender to sleep. Notice their transient nature and the point where you experience yourself truly letting go, or "dying" into sleep.

Obtaining Professional Help

Occasional difficulties in falling asleep are common and usually remit on their own in a short time. If sleep onset difficulties persist, they should be evaluated by a qualified health care professional. Despite failing to acknowledge the spiritual dimensions of sleep problems, most sleep doctors are technically excellent and can provide useful guidance. Some words of advice: be particularly cautious about sleeping pills; if you need to take something, care-fully consider all the alternatives, including complementary and alternative medicine. And be sure to add your own sense of spiri-tuality to the mix.

⌒

The familiar forms and activities of daytime life, including all of the social and visual cues that guide and define us, begin to fade at dusk, threatening to deprive us of our ordinary, waking sense of self. Many of us simply do not know who we are in the dark. So we turn on the lights. It is time we seriously consider losing our naïve, childhood tendencies to fear the dark, to associate darkness with evil. The metaphor is poetic but immature, and it perpetuates our night blindness. As we will see in chapter 8 when we examine shadow, literal darkness is not evil. It is healing.

⌒4

Darkness: Sleep and Serenity

Once there was a way to get back homeward
Once there was a way to get back home
Sleep pretty darling do not cry
And I will sing a lullaby

—THOMAS DEKKER AND
PAUL MCCARTNEY

STAR TREK'S SEVEN-OF-NINE, a hot, rigid, partially rehabili-
tated half-human and half-robotic "Borg," taught a recent generation that incessant drive could still be sexy. She was remarkably
productive, quick, no-nonsense, and highly efficient. Thomas
Edison's kind of gal, I suppose. But despite the distinctly advanced technology of her futuristic era, she still had to endure
the inconvenience of sleep. Or at least of regular "regeneration,"
which she did standing up in an energy pod in Cargo Bay II of the
Starship *Enterprise*.

This is our emerging myth of sleep—it is a mechanistic necessity. Sleep is essentially technical—we regenerate or recharge our
batteries. Nothing personal or meaningful about it. Subjectively,
sleep is experienced as a *knockout*—we go offline, become unconscious, or dead to the world. From a cultural perspective, sleep is
simply inconvenient since it renders us inoperable. Despite much
lip service to the contrary, our behavior suggests that we view sleep
as an annoying necessity. We would much rather be doing something truly productive.

Philosophically, this mechanistic posture strongly informs contemporary culture's view of sleep and underpins our approach to sleep science. Filled with interesting historical, scientific, and practical information, *The Promise of Sleep*, by William Dement, is one of the foremost popular books on sleep available today. Centered on the book's original hardcover jacket is a large, distinct, circular image reminiscent of the inside of a clock. With multiple metal gears, cogs, and wheels, this image reminds us that, ultimately, the promise of sleep is about understanding a complex mechanism—a machine. And although the image suggests a basic regard for rhythm, it is not the gentle ebb and flow of natural rhythms but the incessant clicking of a mechanism—something that has no consciousness, is not sentient, and needs to be managed.

Such a rigid, mechanistic view undermines our sleep health and clouds our personal and spiritual understanding of sleep. When we think of ourselves as hybrids like Seven-of-Nine—half-human and half-machine—we fail to recognize the delicate, subjective, and sacred dimensions to sleep. Our challenge then is to appreciate the mechanisms of sleep without sacrificing its deeply personal and incomparably serene spirit.

Descending into Deep Sleep

In chapter 2 we reviewed the basics of sleep architecture, those rhythmic changes in brain wave activity used by sleep specialists to define night consciousness. We saw that night consciousness is structured by recurring ninety-minute ultradian rhythms, each composed of alternating segments of stage sleep and dreaming. In the previous chapter, we explored the call to surrender associated with Stage 1 and Stage 2 sleep. This chapter will consider Stages 3 and 4 sleep, which are characterized by theta and delta brain wave activity. Collectively referred to as *deep sleep*, we normally experience most of this profoundly restful, "slow wave" sleep in the first half of the night—during the descent of darkness.

Deep sleep is the internal representation of the descent of night. To enter and sustain deep sleep we must be willing to be like the night—we must be willing to slow, to allow the mind to quiet and the body to cool. Attaining deep sleep is essentially about resonating with the slow and spacious rhythms of night.

As sleep progressively deepens, our thinking virtually stops, respiration becomes slow and regular, cardiovascular activity eases, and our muscles relax. Closed to the public, the body and brain now shift into maintenance mode. Nyx continues ascending the summit of the night sky, cooling the earth below, while our melatonin levels also continue to climb, cooling the body. In deep sleep we are about as cool and still as we can get this side of death. It is fitting, once again, that Thanatos, the Greek god of death, is the twin brother of Hypnos. Compared to waking, in deep sleep we are dead to the world. But, if we are, indeed, dead to the world, could it be that we come to life elsewhere?

As we finish our day's waking in the world, we are ushered home by night. Home is our foundation, a safe place for respite and an opportunity for rejuvenation. As the outer world dissolves into night, we are whisked deeply into our interiors, home to a sacred sense of ourselves. Sleep is, indeed, remarkably rejuvenating to body and soul. It is a place of respite that is at the same time powerfully healing and profoundly serene. As the opening lullaby suggests, we might come to remember sleep as *a way to get back home.*

Deep Sleep and Health

Obtaining sufficient deep sleep is arguably one of the most important things we can do to optimize our health. Our bodies and brains depend heavily upon it. Selectively depriving research subjects of deep sleep eventually results in its rebounding with force. Animals continuously deprived of deep sleep will grow ill and die within a few weeks.

The increasing levels of melatonin accompanying deep sleep promote immune activity, protect us from viral infections, and have remarkable anticancerous properties. Deep sleep is also linked to the production of human growth hormone (HGH), which is instrumental in a broad range of important biological processes, including the cellular absorption of nutrients, enhanced immunity, and the maintenance of healthy weight, lean muscle mass, and stamina.

Young adults deprived of deep sleep over several nights were found to have quickly developed symptoms commonly associated with chronic fatigue and fibromyalgia syndrome. In a related study, men who were deprived of half of their regular nightly sleep suffered more than a 25 percent decrease in immune function of natural killer cells on the following day. Regularly missing a few hours of sleep per night may also be associated with increases in heart disease. Sleep deprivation has been linked to heightened levels of inflammatory markers known as cytokines and C-reactive protein, both associated with increased cardiovascular risk.

According to recent findings, deep sleep plays a critical role in maintaining normal body weight. Sleep deprivation studies involving healthy young men resulted in significant increases in the hormones leptin and cortisol, both involved in the regulation of hunger. Sleep loss was also associated with impaired glucose tolerance, a prediabetic state that, fortunately, returned to normal with adequate sleep. People whose deep sleep is compromised by sleep apnea, a serious obstruction of breathing during sleep, have also been found to have impaired glucose tolerance. As a group, these people are generally overweight as well. It is interesting to note that the rise in obesity in the United States over recent decades appears to be correlated with a drop in our average sleep length and progressive increases in LAN.

Unfortunately, most of us will experience a significant loss of deep sleep as we age. Men under the age of twenty-five normally spend about 20 percent of their total sleep time in deep sleep. By the time they are thirty-five, only about 5 percent of their total sleep time is spent in deep sleep. This drop is associated with a 75 percent decrease in HGH. By the age of fifty most men seem to have virtually lost the capacity to experience deep sleep and are producing only negligible amounts of HGH. Unfortunately, men over fifty were also found to have elevated nighttime levels of cortisol, which is associated with fragmented sleep, memory difficulties, and a heightened predisposition to diabetes.

There is widespread belief today that sleep quantity and quality normally diminish with age. But it may be the other way around; that is, we prematurely age as a result of chronically poor sleep. Recent research suggests that the common signs of what we consider normal aging may, in fact, be symptoms of chronic sleep deprivation. Growing evidence suggests that many of the physiological as well as psychological decrements typically associated with aging may actually result from chronic sleep loss.

As people age, they are also more likely to use medications, many of which can compromise sleep. Beta-blockers, for example, can inhibit melatonin production in the brain. Aspirin and other NSAIDs (nonsteroidal anti-inflammatory drugs), diuretics, and benzodiazepine tranquilizers also suppress melatonin. From sleeping pills to psychiatric medications and painkillers, many other commonly used medicines also disrupt our circadian rhythms, further compromising sleep and dreams.

I believe that many sleep problems among the elderly may be less related to age per se, and more the result of lifestyle—*how* we age in our culture. Our chronic overexposure to LAN, excessive sleeping pill and substance use, and the long-term impact of overly driven lifestyles are all likely factors in the degradation of our sleep over time.

Fortunately for women, they generally obtain more deep sleep than men. On average, men get about forty minutes of deep sleep per night while women get about seventy minutes. Some experts believe this may be nature's attempt to compensate for sleep loss associated with caring for infants. Whatever the cause, it may be linked to the fact that women tend to outlive men by an average of seven years.

Although there is no consensus among sleep specialists about exactly how much sleep we need each night, there is general agreement that it is in the neighborhood of seven to nine hours for adults. Some people seem to get by with less, while others may need more. There is, however, widespread agreement that as a society we are not obtaining sufficient sleep. Unfortunately, obtaining sufficient sleep is not a guarantee that we are getting good sleep. Quantity does not assure quality. Whether the result of insufficient sleep or compromised sleep quality, inadequate deep sleep can make us sick, fat, and old beyond our years. Maybe this is the only recourse Mother Nature has to try to get some of us to slow down, rest, and come home to sleep.

Deep Sleep Disturbances

Our deep sleep is badly damaged. It is woefully insufficient and seriously fragmented. Most obviously, it is compromised by insomnias and disrupted by a host of other medical disorders like sleep apnea, limb movement disorders, and digestive reflux. In the middle of the night, millions of us routinely lie awake tossing and turning. While many people know that their deep sleep is disturbed and unrefreshing, many millions more are losing quality sleep and not even aware of it. They believe they are asleep but ache, kick, choke, and nearly suffocate their way through the night, never venturing beyond the lighter stages of sleep. Hard-pressed to explain their excessive daytime sleepiness, they commonly mask this symptom with stimulating substances, overeating, or frenetic activity.

Sleep Maintenance Insomnia

After falling asleep, tens of millions of us regularly struggle with staying asleep through the night—with sleep maintenance insomnia. According to the National Sleep Foundation (2005), 32 percent of American adults report waking up repeatedly during the night at least a few nights each week. Twenty-four percent struggle with early morning awakenings from which they are unable to get back to sleep. And 38 percent of American adults report awakening unrefreshed at least a few days each week—presumably the result of fragmented or nonrestorative sleep that they may be completely unaware of.

Virtually everyone has experienced an occasional night or short course of sleep maintenance insomnia. For many, however, middle-of-the-night sleeplessness becomes a chronic struggle that can persist for years and even decades. And, insomnia is usually a quiet, private, and lonely struggle. There is little comfort in the large numbers of those who share in the ordeal. For most, the anguish of being unable to sleep at night is further complicated by anxieties about remaining alert by day. And knowing that this anguish and anxiety only exacerbate insomnia frequently results in even more anguish and anxiety. As one of my insomnia patients, Matthew, a mid-forties, successful, and highly-stressed business executive, blatantly states, "It's a dirty trick."

People who have occasional, infrequent awakenings generally seem to take it in stride. They understand that the problem will resolve and are confident that they will soon return to a normal sleeping pattern. Seasoned insomniacs like Matthew, however, commonly develop a damaging pattern of reactions that perpetuates their nighttime awakenings.

Matthew came to see me after struggling with frequent middle-of-the-night awakenings for nearly two years. He had tried a course of prescription sleeping pills, which helped initially but later lost its effectiveness. Concerned that his compromised sleep was affecting the quality of his work, Matthew became increasingly anxious at night.

"So what happens when you first awaken and realize that it's still the middle of the night?" I asked.

"Well, nothing, really. I toss and turn. I check the time and eventually I get up to pee and I—"

"No, Matthew," I interrupted. "I mean what happens *inside your head* when you first awaken? What thoughts cross your mind?"

"Hmm." He reflected on my question for a few seconds. "You really want to know?"

"Yes, of course," I said.

"Well, I know exactly what happens," Matthew continued. "I think . . . *oh shit!*"

In my experience, variations of this kind of internal reaction to insomnia are quite common. We often greet our middle-of-the-night awakenings with expletives and rousing emotion. This is no surprise given the tremendous frustration associated with such awakenings, but it simply worsens the problem. In chapter 3 we saw that bedtime prayers or blessings were useful in facilitating healthy sleep onset. I think it is safe to assume that bedtime curses will have the opposite effect on sleep maintenance. Unfortunately, these common reactions only throw more fuel on the fire of our wakefulness. And the resulting smoke makes it difficult to determine what is really disrupting our sleep.

Determining exactly what compromises the quality of deep sleep may appear to be a simple matter, but it is not. Many people, for example, believe that their bladders awaken them in the middle of the night. Most sleep specialists, however, do not agree. It is probable that we first awaken and then notice our bothersome bladder, blaming it for waking us up. Most of us are familiar with the experience of sleeping through the night to awaken in the morning with a bulging bladder. Often, the bladder we blame for waking us is not even near our capacity.

Likewise, we may conclude that things like occasional hot flashes, minor muscle aches, some slight hunger, or our partner's light snoring is waking us up. As is most evident with cognitive popcorn, the things we notice upon awakening are not necessarily the things that cause our awakenings. But if cognitive popcorn, other minor discomforts, and bothersome bladders do not put us over the top, then what does? What awakens us in the middle of the night?

In principle, I believe we awaken primarily because we have not ventured deeply enough into sleep. We remain too anxious to completely let go, hovering close to the surface of our waking consciousness. If sleep is a homecoming, we do not make it all the way there. We get waylaid by the unfinished business of our waking minds and unresolved discomfort in our bodies. Earlier we saw that sleep requires that our *bodies cool, our minds quiet, and our clocks slow.* Unfortunately, millions of us try to sleep with perpetually *noisy minds, runaway personal clocks,* and chronic *bodily inflammation.*

Noisy Minds

Just as repressed and denied daytime issues can impair sleep onset, I believe they can later disrupt the maintenance of our deep sleep. Cognitive popcorn can occur as readily in the middle of the night as it does at the start of sleep. This popping is symptomatic of underlying anxiety—a noisy mind.

There is a common belief that if a noisy mind does not prevent us from falling asleep at the beginning of the night, it will not awaken us later. This is not true. The stimulation of even a very noisy mind can be masked by excessive sleepiness, allowing us to fall asleep at the beginning of the night. But as the weight of our sleepiness gradually diminishes with sleep attained, underlying noise can emerge and wake us up.

In contrast to sleep onset problems, which are usually associated with anxiety, middle-of-the-night mind noise has been linked to depression. This is particularly true as we get older. We will look more closely at the relationship of depression to sleep maintenance insomnia in the following chapter when we discuss dreaming.

As we age, there is also a common tendency to awaken much too early in the morning and experience difficulty returning to sleep. When this is not the result of an underlying noisy mind, it can be symptomatic of an advanced sleep phase—what we might think of as a *quick clock.*

Quick Clocks

Throughout our early and mid-adult years the inertia of our speedy subjective clocks makes it hard to slow down, let go, and sleep at day's end. We too frequently overrun our bedtime with activity and then cannot slow our buzzing minds sufficiently to fall asleep. I have come to wonder if a lifetime of chronic hurriedness might permanently speed up our personal clocks.

We saw previously that as we age, our personal clocks do seem to speed up, increasing the likelihood of an advanced sleep phase. A clock that runs fast will, of course, tell us that it is actually later than it really is. When our personal clocks run fast, they may inform us that it is bedtime hours before it actually is. Whether we go to bed at the prompting of our fast clocks or not, they will, likewise, awaken us hours before our normal rising time.

We might also think about our personal clocks in a more qualitative way. Our body clocks do not simply tell time; they also mete out ultradian rhythms, providing a framework of *timing* for our psychological and biological functioning. Disruptions of our personal clocks are also associated with changes in breathing patterns, mood states, psychological and neurological rhythms, as well as appetite and digestive cycles. It is not surprising then that disruptions of our body clocks can compromise the quality of our sleep.

Bodily Inflammation

One of the most promising medical discoveries in recent years has been about the key role of chronic inflammation as an undercurrent in many disease processes. Bodily inflammation appears to be a factor in a wide range of diseases, including heart disease, diabetes, and even cancer. As suggested earlier, compromised deep sleep may be one critical factor in the development of such inflammation. Sleep-related breathing disorders, nighttime limb movements, and digestive reflux are the three most common medical conditions that prevent our bodies from resting and cooling sufficiently to enter and sustain deep sleep.

Breathing difficulties, including snoring and obstructive sleep apnea, are one of the major causes of disrupted sleep. Thirty-two percent of American adults report that they snore at least a few nights a week, according to the National Sleep Foundation (2005).

Of this group, 24 percent stated that they snored every night or almost every night. Men were more likely than women to report snoring, and older adults are also more likely to snore.

Biological factors can predispose one to develop constriction in the airway during sleep, resulting in snoring as one inhales. Simple, or primary snoring, is not as innocuous as it was once thought and can be a risk factor for hypertension and diabetes as well as a symptom of sleep apnea. It can also contribute to fragmented sleep and interfere with the sleep of one's bed partner. Snoring has been linked to headaches, daytime fatigue, and relationship discord. Weight gain, the consumption of alcohol, and smoking are known to significantly exacerbate snoring.

As the airway constriction that causes primary snoring progresses, breathing can become seriously compromised. Obstructive sleep apnea, or OSA, results when breathing repeatedly slows or actually stops for varying intervals throughout the night, resulting in a potentially dangerous drop in blood oxygen levels. This cyclic pattern of suffocation can significantly fragment sleep and diminish if not completely inhibit both deep sleep and dreaming. OSA places tremendous strain on one's cardiovascular system and is commonly associated with weight gain, hypertension, diabetes, and, of course, excessive daytime sleepiness. Strangely enough, since people with OSA usually have amnesia for the repeated arousals that impair their sleep, they might actually believe they are good sleepers. They simply cannot explain why they are so sleepy during the day. Recent estimates suggest that up to 30 million American adults suffer from OSA. The vast majority of these individuals remain undiagnosed and, therefore, untreated.

Nighttime or *periodic limb movements in sleep* (also known as PLMS) are another common cause of nocturnal arousals. PLMS refer to rhythmic movements, usually in the legs, that repeat in twenty- to forty-second cycles during sleep. Characterized by brief muscle twitches or jerky movements involving an upward flexing of the feet, they tend to occur in episodes lasting from a few minutes to a number of hours. Most often, like OSA, people with PLMS are unaware that they have this disorder and remain undiagnosed and untreated. Although they do occur in younger people, more than one-third of adults over the age of sixty-five have PLMS. The specific causes of PLMS remain uncertain, although nervous system or vascular problems are suspected. PLMS are a probable factor in the fragmented sleep of millions of Americans.

An estimated 8 million Americans suffer from digestive or *gastro-esophageal reflux disease* (GERD), a condition in which the contents of the stomach are regurgitated into the esophagus when one is supine. GERD is characterized by awakenings with choking sensations that can be similar to those associated with obstructive sleep apnea. Causes of GERD can include a weakened lower esophageal sphincter, eating hard-to-digest foods, and dysrhythmic eating patterns. When we eat at times that are out of sync with our body clock's expectations, our digestion can become impaired.

OSA, PLMS, and GERD are the three most common medical disorders associated with bodily inflammation and sleep disturbances. As disruptive as they are to deep sleep, these conditions do not usually result in obvious awakenings. They do routinely cause significant and repeated unconscious arousals that compromise sleep quality. And because we are often unaware of them, when they do fully awaken us, we will likely try to attribute the awakening to some other cause.

Although these sleep disorders might appear to be obvious biomedical conditions, they are not without significant behavioral influences. Our behavior, our patterns of eating, activity (or lack thereof), and substance use, for example, commonly exacerbate OSA, PLMS, and GERD, if not directly contribute to their cause. Such patterns of dysfunctional daily living are, furthermore, reflections of how many of us manage our daytime anxieties. This raises a critical question regarding the degree to which such deep sleep disorders may also represent a biological opportunistic emergence of repressed or denied waking anxieties.

Although sleep disorders are defined in terms of complex, specific physiological symptoms, they are ultimately manifestations of minds that will not quiet, clocks that cannot slow, and bodies that do not cool. Beyond addressing any specific medical symptoms we might have, it is critical to also become more aware of our basic relationship with our minds, our bodies, and our personal clocks. We need to determine if we are using the body and the mind as a nighttime dumping ground for daytime troubles. Are we using substances during waking to suppress our emotions? Are we eating inappropriately at night to quell unwanted emotions or loneliness? Are we secretly displacing our unexamined anxieties in our nervous systems or burying denied tensions in our muscles?

Deep Sleep Solutions

"Okay ... we have about thirty seconds left here and I have one last question for you, Dr. Naiman." The interviewer, a man with about four cups of morning coffee coursing through his veins, smiled hard and fast as my brief spot on sleep problems was being broadcast through a number of news radio markets around the country. He had already run through the list of our agreed upon questions and proceeded to ad lib. "So," he continued, "what is *the* secret of a good night's sleep?"

It was the dreaded *magic bullet* question.

"*The* secret of a good ... uh ... night's sleep ..." I stuttered and paused because I simply didn't know what to say.

The assumption that there is a magic bullet, a single, simple solution to multifaceted and complex health problems like sleep disorders is a myth that health professionals generally try to dispel. It is a myth that can interfere with comprehensive and personalized treatment by lulling people into the false hope of a simplistic, impersonal, one-size-fits-all solution. It was a myth I thought I had put to rest in the preceding moments of the interview.

"The secret of a good night's sleep ..." I was frustrated and lapsed into wise-ass mode. "The secret of a good night's sleep," I heard myself say, "... that would be a good day's waking."

Despite championing a comprehensive approach to sleep problems, when it comes to practice, sleep medicine relies heavily on a magic bullet philosophy. The most common treatments for major sleep disorders involve medications and mechanisms—pills for insomnias, PLMS, and GERD, and continuous positive airway pressure (CPAP), a breathing machine for apnea. Such approaches to treatment have an important place in managing the serious symptoms of these conditions, but they are generally stopgap measures that do not address the root of the problems.

A few years ago, Homer Simpson, the acclaimed cartoon icon, was diagnosed with OSA. This perpetually middle-aged, overweight, excessively sleepy fellow snored loudly, loved his donuts and beer, and was regularly nodding off at his job at the Springfield nuclear power plant. We should have known. Homer was treated with CPAP, a breathing-enhancing device hooked to a Darth Vader–like face mask strapped around his head. He could be the poster child for the mechanistic model of sleep medicine. Unfortunately, CPAP is as uncomfortable as it sounds and frequently results in a lack of treatment adherence.

As carefully as sleep doctors may explain the complex factors contributing to OSA to their patients—as much as they may discuss the importance of weight management, encourage exercise, and warn about alcohol and nicotine exacerbating the problem—the emphasis on CPAP treatment gives a different message. The fact that a mechanical device may quickly restore desperately needed sleep suggests that a simple mechanical glitch caused the difficulty in the first place.

Sleeping pills are used not only to compensate for our inability to let go into sleep but also to manage our difficulty with staying asleep. The widespread belief that sleep is mere unconsciousness reinforces the excessive use of magic bullet pills to treat sleep maintenance insomnia. Sleeping pills are not very precise magic bullets. In fact, most are more like the scatter of shotgun pellets that take broad aim at wakefulness but simultaneously hit and damage deep sleep and dreaming in the process. Sleeping pills generally increase lighter, Stage 2 sleep at the cost of deep sleep and dreaming. They may also cause amnesia for awakenings, diminishing frustration but leaving one with a false sense of improved sleep. As I mentioned earlier, sleeping pills can result in habituation and dependence, compromising our natural ability to fall and stay asleep.

In the end, sleeping pills do little more than mask our night-time symptoms of sleeplessness. In contrast to the messages of glitzy television ads, I have never met anyone who awakened refreshed and perky after taking a sleeping pill. Sleeping pills do not restore normal and natural sleep. They merely induce unconsciousness. Unfortunately, many of us do not know how to distinguish between the two. Fortunately, many of us still remain leery about the use of such magic bullet pills.

A National Sleep Foundation poll revealed that less than 10 percent of people with sleep disorders have been diagnosed and an even smaller percentage have been treated (2002). The problem of diagnosing and treating sleep disorders has been attributed to a lack of training on the part of primary care physicians as well as to a serious dearth of sleep doctors. But other data and experience suggest that people are also reluctant to talk about sleep concerns with their doctors. In addition to the millions who regularly use sleeping pills and CPAP machines, millions more are apprehensive about doing so. Believing magic bullets are all they will get from their doctors, they avoid medical care for sleep issues altogether. They trust their instinct that sleep is not unconsciousness and breathing cannot be reduced to a bionic function. They do not want magic bullets.

In principle, I have no argument with the notion of a magic bullet. The judicious use of sleeping pills has a place in treatment, and CPAP devices have unquestionably saved many lives. In fact, I believe there are *many* valuable magic bullets. Witness the dozens of sleep books that offer hundreds of sleep improvement tips, tricks, techniques, and tactics. In recent years the emergence of complementary and alternative medicine (CAM) has broadened these options immensely. Drawing from fields such as clinical nutrition, homeopathic medicine, acupuncture and traditional Chinese medicine, naturopathic medicine, and energy medicine, CAM dramatically expands our options with a broad range of potentially effective sleep aids and strategies.

The main problem with a magic bullet approach is that it attempts to address sleep issues outside of a meaningful, comprehensive context. Having lost the forest for the trees, we take magic bullet potshots at our sleep symptoms. As much as I would prefer a less mechanistic metaphor, what we really need is a kind of *magic gun*—a new conceptual framework for organizing and delivering the broad range of magic bullet interventions. Such a framework must be comprehensive and integrative, taking simultaneous aim at all relevant body, mind, and clock issues. It must be sensitive to all biological, psychological, and other lifestyle factors. It must also offer sensitivity to the role of rhythms and resonance. The secret of a good night's sleep does, indeed, involve all the complexities inherent in a good day's waking. Ultimately, we need to recognize that the vast majority of people with sleep disorders are struggling with lifestyle issues.

As my news interview ended, I unclipped my microphone and began to walk away. The interviewer called to me once again with a big smile on his face.

"So, just one final question, Dr. Naiman. What is the secret of a good day's waking?"

I couldn't resist. "A good night's sleep."

A Good Night's Sleep

Our personal, subjective sense of a good night's sleep is based not on the actual experience of sleep but on amnesia about it. Like dental work or symptoms of the flu, sleep is something we prefer to be largely unaware of. We do not determine our sleep quality directly but by the degree of our unconsciousness of it. For most of us, then, a memorable sleep is one that we cannot remember.

Assuming that good-quality deep sleep is synonymous with unconsciousness can cause us to react with judgment to any awareness we might have during sleep. We presume that virtually all awakenings or any awareness during sleep is problematic. Like Matthew, we are poised to come at our nighttime awareness with expletives and critical cognitions. As an alternative, we might learn to meet them mindfully and with grace.

Sarah was an attractive, feisty, white-haired woman who came to see me a number of years ago to explore her dreams. She had retired a couple of years before and was enjoying a slower-paced life focused on family, gardening, and a deepening interest in personal and spiritual growth. At sixty-two, she was in good physical and mental health and generally happy with her life.

I noticed from the start that Sarah had exceptional dream recall, as evidenced by the number and details of the dreams she regularly recorded. "You seem to have an easy time remembering your dreams," I said to her in our second session.

"I do," she said, smiling. "Especially since I've been able to catch the ones in the middle of the night when I awaken."

"When you awaken in the middle of the night?" I repeated, concerned that she might have insomnia.

"Well, yes," she said. "I think I'm up most nights now for an hour or so—I don't know. I don't really look at the clock."

"Please tell me more about this," I said.

"Well, there's not much to tell," Sarah continued. "After I sleep for about three or four hours, I seem to just slowly drift awake. I know it sounds strange, but it's actually quite pleasant. I'm sort of half-awake and half-asleep and feeling pretty peaceful. My mind is usually quiet and clear. I'll jot down notes from a dream and then just sort of be. I guess I eventually slip back into deeper sleep at some point because I have more dreams." She paused and looked into my eyes. "It's really not a problem," she emphasized, clearly sensing my concern. "I really do get a good night's sleep."

After evaluating her sleep patterns and daytime energy more thoroughly, I concluded that Sarah did not technically suffer from insomnia. Although such experiences of comfortable nightly awakenings are not commonly reported, they are not unheard of. Recent scientific findings and historical research strongly suggest that certain patterns of awakening during nightly sleep may be natural, normal, and, perhaps, even beneficial.

Sleep medicine has long struggled to try to make sense of an odd phenomenon known as *sleep state misperception*. People with this condition report chronic, severe, and often nightlong bouts of insomnia. But despite their repeated subjective experience of nighttime wakefulness, they usually have little, if any, daytime sleepiness. And when they are evaluated in overnight sleep studies, they surprisingly appear to sleep fairly well by standard objective measures. When people with sleep state misperception are given sleeping pills, their sleep may actually worsen by objective measures, but they stop complaining that they are awake. They get knocked out.

Sleep state misperception may actually represent spontaneous experiences of awareness during sleep. Is it possible that sleep state misperception is actually a form of *sleep state perception*? Could it be that some kinds of nighttime awakenings or awareness during sleep are normal? Perhaps it is time that we reconsider our notions of normal sleep.

By common definition, sleeping and waking are mutually exclusive states. But, as Sarah's experience reflects, sleeping and awareness are not. Odd as it sounds, a number of studies suggest that we are fully capable of being aware during sleep.

Specific brain wave changes that typically occur in Stage 2 sleep are considered to be the criterion for the onset of true sleep. Despite this, good sleepers who are roused out of Stage 2 sleep will report that they were already awake more than half the time. (Under similar circumstances, about 80 percent of insomniacs will report that they were already awake.) We have seen that, collectively, Stage 3 and 4 sleep is considered the deepest possible level of sleep. Interestingly, 5 percent of good sleepers reaching deep sleep during a nap reported that they were still awake.

Night Watch

Dr. Thomas A. Wehr conducted a study (1999) to gain some insight into natural sleep patterns prior to the use of excessive nighttime illumination. He found that when healthy adults were prohibited from using artificial light at night—from dusk until dawn—their sleep patterns went through an unusual transformation. People who previously slept in standard consolidated blocks of time eventually began sleeping in two distinct periods separated by an hour or so of wakeful deep rest and reflection.

Participants in Wehr's study developed a curious pattern of lying comfortably awake for an hour or more before falling asleep, sleeping deeply for a few hours, awakening in peaceful contemplation for an hour or more, and then returning to sleep for a few more hours. Wehr found that during their comfortable periods of wakefulness his subjects had elevated levels of prolactin, a hormone associated with deep repose. He believes that overexposure to artificial light may diminish prolactin by distorting natural circadian rhythms.

This research raises the question of whether all nightly awakenings are, in fact, appropriately labeled as insomnia. Wehr believes that some of these awakenings may be characteristic of a more natural human sleep pattern reemerging in an unreceptive world. He speculates that the lack of waking time in darkness deprives modern people of natural, regular periods of spiritual reflection and contemplation.

Dr. A. Roger Ekirch's extensive study (2005) of night behavior and sleep patterns of the preindustrial era sheds further light on what might constitute a more natural sleep pattern. Ekirch found that the sleep of preindustrial people occurred in two distinct phases identical to those observed by Wehr. People typically spent three or four hours in what was called a "first sleep" and then awakened to a "night watch." This hour or two of darkened awareness presented interesting opportunities for a kind of nightlife that we have since lost. People typically remained in bed to meditate or pray, reflect on the day, converse and make love with their partners, and consider their dreams, which were frequently used to guide their waking lives. It was not uncommon for people to allow their minds to wander into a special kind of reverie—a highly valued altered state of consciousness. A "second" or "morning" sleep of three or four hours then followed this night watch.

Disregard for the subjective experiences associated with sleep is one of the most damaging consequences of our night blindness. Such a perspective pathologizes virtually all nighttime awakenings and awareness as insomnia, discouraging us from more deeply accessing night consciousness. Is it possible that at least some of what we consider insomnia today might be better understood as a vestige of a natural, biphasic sleep pattern? Could middle-of-the-night awakenings be the light center of the dark wave in the yin-yang symbol? Might a greater lucidity around sleep be a passageway to serenity?

Sarah found it difficult to describe her middle-of-the-night experience of awakening in words. It was a half-sleep and half-awake state, a kind of hybrid consciousness most of us are not familiar with—a way of being that is dismissed by our waking world. Are we awake, asleep, or somewhere in between during such a watching period?

Opening to lucid sleep might help us reconceptualize our limiting medical notions of insomnia. Sarah's spontaneous experiences of peaceful nightly awakenings cannot reasonably be classified as insomnia. Such nightly awakenings and awareness seem to be part of a more natural human sleep pattern. When we judge all awakenings as problematic, we engage in struggles to get back to sleep and overlook what could be a personal spiritual opportunity. After working with many individuals who have had experiences similar to Sarah's, I am no longer quick to judge all nighttime wakefulness as pathological.

In recent years, philosophers and psychologists engaged in consciousness studies are beginning to offer further reflections on this question. They are coming to concur with ancient yogic and other spiritual teachings about the possibility of cultivating lucidity during deep sleep. It is in our deepest sleep that we discover one of spirituality's greatest paradoxes: sleeping and waking are not opposite and mutually exclusive states of consciousness. "Sleep lingers all our lifetime about our eyes, as night hovers all day in the boughs of the fir tree," wrote Ralph Waldo Emerson.

Sleep as a Spiritual Practice

From a mechanistic perspective, there is no question about what we experience subjectively in our deep sleep. *Nothing*. Dr. William Dement makes this point clear in *The Promise of Sleep*: "We never know we're sleeping while we're asleep. It is impossible to have conscious, experiential knowledge of non-dreaming sleep; indeed, one of sleep's defining aspects is that we don't know that we are sleeping while we are doing it" (1999, 14).

In sharp contrast, a number of mystical and spiritual traditions teach that awareness during sleep is both a feasible and desirable goal. Yoga Nidra techniques derived from Hinduism guide practitioners into experiencing a form of waking sleep. Likewise, Tibetan Buddhism has evolved elaborate and challenging meditative practices designed specifically to cultivate awareness during sleep. "Sleep," says the Dalai Lama, "is the best meditation." Tibetan Buddhist sleep and dream yoga teaches practitioners to literally witness sleep. And what is it that they might witness? *Nothing.*

Research has determined that advanced meditation practitioners were more likely to report spontaneous awareness during deep sleep. Accessing deeply relaxed states of consciousness during meditation, including theta and delta states, allows practitioners to become familiar with and subsequently be able to identify these same states during sleep. Through such practices, they develop a frame of reference for that profoundly serene nothingness. In contrast to the Western world where the notion of "nothing" connotes a lack of value, in Eastern thinking, nothing or emptiness is the sacred source of everything. It is synonymous with serenity.

Lucid sleep is the simple and spiritually elegant awareness of awareness itself. It is pure awareness—independent of any objects of awareness. Stephen Levine teaches that what we are all really looking for is the part of us doing the looking. This part becomes especially visible in deep sleep.

Learning to cultivate awareness during deep sleep is a challenging but also rewarding spiritual practice. The practice of lucid sleep offers benefits comparable to the deepest meditation, a profound serenity available to all. But even if lucid sleeping is a potential we all may be able to realize, why would one want to? If I am resting quietly in deep sleep, why would I want to be conscious of it?

In a spiritual sense, we are more our true selves, closer to who we really are, at home in deep sleep. It is a time of perfect stillness and immeasurable serenity. Because there is nothing, there is nothing to judge, so we can experience being completely nonjudgmental in deep sleep. In cultivating conscious experiences of this state of deep serenity, we can better learn its coordinates and more readily access it during waking.

Lucid Sleep Practices

Truly healing our sleep requires that we become mindful of the full range of body, mind, and clock factors that influence our nights. The following practices are offered to help you better understand and open to experiencing deep sleep.

Address Disruptive Body, Mind, and Clock Factors

Remain mindful of the important link between lifestyle and deep sleep. Consider how all aspects of your lifestyle affect your body, mind, and clock and its relationship to your sleep quantity and quality. If you suspect that you have a medical sleep disorder like PLMS, GERD, or sleep apnea, please address these concerns with a qualified physician.

Maintaining good general physical health, including adequate nutrition, regular exercise, and a sensible posture toward substances will support your body in cooling at night.

If you experience occasional difficulty in returning to sleep from middle-of-the-night awakenings, use the cognitive popcorn exercise described at the end of chapter 3. Allow yourself to "unpack" and explore any automatic reactions you might have to middle-of-the-night awakenings. Notice if you greet these with judgmental expletives or gentle receptivity. Try to understand the underlying appraisals you make of these awakenings. What are you telling yourself about them? And how might this appraisal affect both the experience of awakening and your ability to return to sleep?

Increase Your Sleep Sensitivity

Increase your personal and social sensitivity to sleep. Ask people in your life about how they sleep. The next time someone asks you about your sleep, consider your reply more thoughtfully. Think and talk about the quality of your sleep. Make it important.

Not all middle-of-the-night awakenings are necessarily indications of insomnia. And even when they are, not all aspects of being awake need be troublesome. Practice being mindful during nighttime awakenings. You might even consider experimenting with intentionally staying awake at night for a few moments after arising to urinate or to get a drink of water. Try lying awake with your eyes open or closed, allowing yourself to experience the deep silence and serenity. If your partner is willing, consider experimenting with the kind of preindustrial nightlife activities mentioned earlier.

Practice Meditation

If you do not already do so, consider starting a daily meditation practice. Mindfulness meditations are particularly adaptable to Western lifestyles and useful in promoting healthy sleep. Yoga Nidra practices that teach a form of lucid sleep are also useful in this regard.

Consider Professional Help

Occasional difficulties in staying asleep are not uncommon and often remit on their own in a short time. If sleep maintenance difficulties persist, however, they should be evaluated by a qualified health care professional with a background in sleep disorders. If you are unaware of symptoms of disrupted deep sleep but remain consistently sleepy during the day, you should also consult with a physician. Carefully consider all of your options, including integrative medicine and complementary and alternative approaches.

~

Sleep pretty darling do not cry
And I will sing a lullaby

A good night's sleep is about a good day's waking. It is a lifestyle issue. And one that is frequently at odds with contemporary culture. It makes sense that a culture with such a warped regard for productivity would fail to acknowledge the spiritual potential of deep sleep, seeing it only as a knockout. The term *lullaby* is derived from the combination of the Old English word *lull,* meaning to hush or call to sleep, and *bye,* the root of *good-bye,* a contraction for *God be with ye.* Deep sleep is a nightly homecoming, a gracious call to serenity.

⁓5

Dreams: Dreaming Dreamers

What dreaming does is give us the fluidity to enter into other worlds by destroying our sense of knowing this world.

—CARLOS CASTANEDA

WHEN WE DREAM, WE BELIEVE WE ARE AWAKE. That is, we usually experience dreaming the same way we do waking—as reality. The only other time we believe we are awake is—well, when we are actually awake. Dreams challenge our fundamental, consensual frame of reality.

I believe this is the main reason we hold our dreams in such limited regard, why we so frequently depersonalize and dismiss them. "It was only a dream" is common advice we might receive from a loved one or a friend, "Just forget it." Because it is only a dream, something unreal, intangible, and essentially inconsequential, we try to forget it. Contemporary sleep science largely supports this stance by viewing dreams as epiphenomena of neural housekeeping functions. Dreams are nothing more than dust clouds stirred by the brain's nightly sweep up. They are meaningless.

But then there is the occasional "big" dream, sometimes nightmarish, often just compelling, eerie, or numinous. A big dream is too large in its scope and depth, much too big emotionally or spiritually to be easily dismissed. Big dreams are gripping. They often linger throughout the day, with residual feelings, with mystery, and with possibility. Big dreams are universal; they visit all people across time and cultures. And big dreams nag at us. They beg for interpretation.

"Let's see. It's dark, night, I guess. I'm sitting on a dirt floor in the stall of an old smelly barn. There's dry manure all around me. It's really dirty. And, it's really kind of eerie. The whole barn feels like it's unstable, like it's coming apart." Marie was reticent to describe the dream she had the night before. As a stressed young mother and full-time university student struggling with depression, she did not have time for dreams. But for reasons she could not explain, she was unable to shake this one. It was a bad dream. A nightmare. A big dream.

Dreams are a superb medium for the expression of shadow issues. Extensive studies of dream content have confirmed that two of every three dreams are, in fact, bad dreams. Schools of depth psychology generally concur in explaining these in terms of compensation for waking repression. Because our ordinary, waking sense of self is usually "asleep" during dreams, its defenses are down. Couple this with the highly malleable reality of the dreamscape and we have an ideal medium for the emergence of our shadows.

"It was really scary." Marie continued. "I . . . I'm leaning against this old splintering wooden partition in the stall. . . . And there's this large, powerful black stallion in the next stall. And he's just kicking and kicking. He's pounding really hard against the partition I'm leaning against and I can't . . . and I realize that I just can't move. I'm really wanting to get up and run but I feel so heavy. I'm scared to death—but it's like I'm paralyzed!"

During dreaming, also referred to as REM, or rapid eye movement sleep, a neurochemical transaction at the center of the brain essentially inhibits our voluntary muscles. With the exception of the muscles that control eye movement, virtually all of our voluntary muscles, the ones we use to move or speak with, become temporarily paralyzed. This *REM atonia* (loss of muscle tone), or *sleep paralysis,* as it is commonly called, is the biological hallmark of dreaming. From a functional perspective, this loss of muscle tone inhibits any movement around or expression of the content of a dream. As we will see, it also has a critical role in processing and healing emotion. When Marie wanted to flee, she encountered her sleep paralysis as a sense of heaviness that further intensified her fear.

"The horse is shrill and angry. It just keeps kicking. . . . I . . . I . . . can feel the wooden partition I'm leaning against starting to crack and splinter." Marie held back her breath, her tears, and her abject fear. "I'm petrified . . . I know . . . I feel like I'm about to die!"

Dreaming teaches us about a fascinating relationship between emotion and motion, between our feelings and movement. The word *motion* lies at the root of the word *emotion*. Interestingly, the nervous system pathways that control our voluntary muscles are rooted in the emotional center of the brain. Emotional energies in the brain generally flow into our muscles, resulting in a proclivity to move. Whether or not we choose to express emotions through some form of motion, we commonly say that we are moved by something that we feel strongly about. When the flow of emotional energy from the brain to our muscles is inhibited by sleep paralysis, our emotions cannot be expressed and discharged into the waking world. Depending on the intensity of the dream, we may experience a powerful backwash of emotional energies reverberating within us, untempered by expression, raw and shadowy.

"Then, I sense myself gradually waking up. Part of me is so relieved as I realize I'm sleeping and it's just a dream. But, it's strange, as terrifying as it was, part of me is still curious about what the horse might do. When I actually awaken, I'm drenched with sweat, and my heart is still pounding like the whole thing was real . . . like it really happened."

All of our dreams, recalled or not, seem to register with the mind and body, much like real events. Our brains buzz, our hearts pound, and our hormones surge in response to dream events, virtually the same way they would to similar waking experiences. Whether or not we are aware of them or remember them, dreams affect us in much the same way our waking experiences do. They are indelibly imprinted in our memories and our cells and on our personalities.

Despite a clear sense that her dream contained important meaning, Marie was ambivalent about discussing it. Because it was charged with terror, she instinctively believed her dream concealed a dire message. "Maybe it's a sign?" she wondered. Marie struggled for some reconciliation with her overpowering dream. When dreams get "big," they cannot be easily dismissed. We feel compelled to interpret and understand them.

"I've always been a bit skittish about horses," Marie admitted. "I think it's a sign that I should just stay where I am."

"Stay where you are?" I wondered.

"Well, you know, I've been incredibly stressed-out for the past year," Marie continued. "The divorce, going back to school, raising my little girl alone, and working nights . . . I felt so boxed in. About a month ago I started fantasizing about getting a place on the outskirts of town. In the country. You know how much I love nature and open spaces. I thought it would help ease the stress."

"And you think the dream might be a sign that you shouldn't move to the country?" I asked.

"Well, I once read an article on dream analysis that said dark things always signified something bad or even evil. That horse was black—as dark as it gets. And dangerous . . . I mean it nearly killed me. It was angry and wild and out of control . . . and, well . . . there are horses in the country." Marie's tone became matter of fact. "That's got to be a bad sign—I know it's a bad omen."

The most common approach to dream interpretation is known as the *dictionary approach*. This perspective suggests that dream images are like words; they have meanings that can be objectively defined. An apple, for example, might symbolize sex. A flower might represent, well, sex again. And a telephone pole would likely represent . . . communication (or maybe in this day and age, phone sex). Beyond this Freudian caricature, much of the world's dream interpretation literature utilizes local variations of a dictionary approach.

The dictionary approach defines images from the dream world in terms of the waking world. Assigning waking world meaning to dream images, whether positive or negative, is comforting in that it provides us with a sense of understanding and control over our dreams. The dream, then, is approached in much the same way that we approach the waking world—with an eye for what is meaningful in the waking world. Because the dictionary approach can help us tame big dreams, even people who are not familiar with it instinctively apply it to their dreams. And this is how Marie approached her nightmare.

Although the dictionary approach is widely used, it depersonalizes our dreams by disregarding their emotional content and personal meaning. In contrast, most formal psychological approaches to dream interpretation do regard the personal emotion and meaning of dream images.

I asked Marie to reconsider the dream from a *gestalt* perspective, which encourages greater personalization of the dream. More specifically, I asked her to retell the dream but to do so from the shadowy perspective of the horse. With a bit of reticence, Marie proceeded. "OK . . . I'm this horse. I'm really dark, black, and I'm muscular and very powerful. And, I'm angry! I'm stuck in this dilapidated barn, confined in this tight little stall. I feel so boxed in. I can't stand it." Marie's eyes grew wide. "I'm kicking and kicking! I want to break out, damn it! I want to be free! I want to run and play in wide-open spaces! I want to be back in nature, in the country!"

Marie burst into tears as she realized that the horse was, in fact, a repressed shadowy aspect of her own self. I was struck, watching her as she spoke, by the fact that she had a dark complexion, was muscular, and, of course, was feeling boxed in by her life. Marie glimpsed the truth of Pogo's *We have met the enemy, and he is us.* She encountered her shadow—a wild, dark, frightening, and even evil image, which, on closer examination, quickly resolved into a passionate and positive messenger from her unconscious. As Marie personalized her dream, its nightmarish angst transformed to excitement about the vision of a new life with much greater freedom.

Marie left with a bold resolve to enact the changes in her life she had so desired. In the days to come, however, the dream's message was gradually trumped by the unremitting demands and incessant drive of her waking—her real life. Despite her momentous insight, Marie was not able to honor the call of her dream. Big as her black stallion nightmare was, it was still just a dream. And as personal and meaningful as its message was, the dream's potency quickly faded when exposed to the light of day.

Dream Deprivation

We live in a world that has little regard for dreams, dreaming, and dreamers. Like his father, Hypnos, and grandmother, Nyx, Morpheus, the Greek god of dreams, is shunned in modern life. There are few places in contemporary culture, especially in the world of sleep science, that truly respect and encourage our dream lives. Many people believe that they only rarely or actually never dream. Others are aware that they dream but only infrequently remember their dreams. In reality, we all dream and normally do so four or five times every night. We do not remember our dreams, however, simply because we do not value, attend to, and understand them. At best, we look at dreams the same way we do stars: they come out at night; we know they are magnificent, but they are far too distant to be of any relevance to our real, waking lives.

Even though not identified as such, many sleep disorders are also dream disorders. Epidemic levels of sleep maintenance insomnia and obstructive sleep apnea probably do as much damage to our dreaming as they do to our sleep. Millions of people with these conditions are routinely aroused or awakened as they enter REM sleep, short-circuiting the experience of dreaming.

To complicate matters, many commonly used medications and substances also suppress REM sleep. Because melatonin mediates dreaming, anything that interferes with normal melatonin production can suppress REM. Ironically, this is true of many prescription and over-the-counter sleeping pills. Sedating antidepressants and minor tranquilizers that are commonly used as sleeping pills, for example, measurably diminish dream sleep. Virtually all antidepressants, now among the most widely prescribed medications, significantly suppress dreaming. NSAIDs, including aspirin, beta blockers, and diuretics suppress melatonin, and, therefore, dreaming.

Likewise, even moderate evening alcohol consumption can interfere with dreaming. As the sedative effects of alcohol wear off,
rebound arousals or awakenings occur at the onset of REM sleep,
short-circuiting the process. Alcohol and nicotine also suppress
melatonin, further depriving us of healthy dreaming.

Largely restricted to the study of the mechanics of REM physi-
ology, conventional sleep medicine virtually ignores the epidemic
of dream deprivation. I have long been baffled at the common tendency for sleep doctors to show little or no concern when people
are dream deprived. As I suggested earlier, contemporary sleep
science boldly dismisses the subjective experience of dreaming as
being meaningless. I believe the widespread thoughtless use of
many common medications with REM-suppressive side effects is
among modern medicine's greatest blunders.

We need to dream. The experimental inhibition of REM sleep
in both animals and humans consistently results in a pressured
REM rebound. This holds true for people whether their dreaming
is limited by sleep disorders or by dream-suppressive medications.
In extreme cases, repressed and damaged dreaming can bounce
back with a vengeance, tearing through the boundary of waking
consciousness as delusions and hallucinations, sudden intrusions
of sleep paralysis, or the literal acting out of dreams as they occur.
Most commonly, however, suppressed dreaming rebounds in a
more subtle and pernicious way, affecting body and mind, health
and mood.

When we are sleep deprived, we become excessively sleepy. Likewise, when we are dream deprived, we become excessively dreamy—
not in any romantic sense, but pathologically so. Because dream
deprivation and sleep deprivation usually overlap, it is difficult to
segregate their effects. I believe, however, that many of the symptoms typically attributed to sleep deprivation are actually symptoms
of dream deprivation.

It makes sense that sleepiness, the unmistakable heavy-headed
proclivity to nod off, results from sleep deprivation. But the dis-
tractibility, concentration difficulties, and perceptual distortions
commonly attributed to being sleepy may be more characteristic of

being dream deprived. Sleepiness is objectively measured by determining how quickly a person will fall asleep when given the opportunity. Studies that selectively deprive people of dreaming for brief periods, however, have found no increase in their objective measures of sleepiness. My clinical experience and recent research suggest that people with chronic dream deprivation are generally less sleepy but probably more fatigued.

In contrast to heavy-headed sleepiness, fatigue is more of a heavy-bodied experience. While the mind may remain alert when we feel fatigued, our muscles are weak and wilted, reminiscent of sleep paralysis. Certain kinds of fatigue may, in fact, represent a subtle rebound of repressed sleep paralysis. Fatigue, like sleep paralysis, wants to limit our ability to discharge emotion through movement. In an effort to compensate for dream suppression, the body attempts to draw us from the extraverted world of waking activity to the shunned and forgotten introverted world of the dream.

Dream Deprivation and Depression

Depression has long been understood in terms of a figurative loss of one's dreams. Although depression is associated with excessive sleepiness, recent studies suggest that depressed individuals may, in fact, be significantly more fatigued than sleepy. Is it possible that depression is also associated with a literal loss of one's dreams, with dream deprivation?

Depression is strongly correlated with sleep maintenance insomnia as well as obstructive sleep apnea, two disorders known to diminish dreaming. Although insomnia is a classic symptom of depression, more recent research indicates it is also an important risk factor for depression. Extended periods of insomnia associated with diminished dreaming significantly increase one's chance of becoming clinically depressed. In fact, a year of insomnia is the single strongest predictor of future clinical depression. Since obstructive sleep apnea can severely suppress dreaming, sometimes resulting in its complete elimination, it is not a surprise that this condition is also strongly correlated with depression.

The discontinuation of dream-suppressive medications or substances is known to result in an acute REM rebound. The backlog of dreams is under pressure to return. Such REM rebounds are usually characterized by a *reduced REM latency*—the premature appearance of dreaming in the nightly sleep cycle. Interestingly, the sleep and dream pattern of depressed individuals is also characterized by a reduced REM latency. Because rebounding dreaming can displace Stage sleep, which normally occupies the first part of the night, depression can leave us both dream and sleep deprived.

Conventional psychiatry looks upon depressive dream rebounds as just another symptom that needs to be treated. It is not surprising, once again, that almost all prescription antidepressant medications significantly reduce REM sleep, further suppressing our dreams as if they were infectious agents. In fact, conventional psychiatry holds that REM suppression may be a key pharmacological mechanism of antidepressant drugs.

REM suppressive antidepressant medications can help restore normal sleep to the first part of the night and thereby reduce daytime sleepiness. But this is accomplished only at the cost of further dream loss. The relief we feel is probably comparable to that obtained when we take medication to reduce a fever.

It should be noted that some people taking antidepressant medications actually report a heightened awareness of dreams. This is not the result of increased REM sleep but of a further increase in REM pressure associated with the constricted flow of dream material. Steeped in a symptom-suppression philosophy, conventional medicine fails to distinguish the baby from the bathwater when it comes to dreaming and depression.

In addition to being offered stimulating antidepressants, depressed individuals are also encouraged by well-meaning family members, friends, and health professionals to get back into gear and get moving. To push past their fatigue. Although addressing the complexities of the treatment of depression is beyond the scope of this work, I do believe that we need to give significantly more consideration to the role of fatigue as a call to heal our dreaming.

Mounting evidence suggests that depressed individuals generally do not dream as richly or deeply as those who are not depressed. Other studies show that dreaming more deeply and richly and remembering one's dreams are useful in healing depression.

Earlier I suggested that being depressed might be more accurately viewed as a need for deep rest. Fatigue may be a kind of mood fever that functions to excuse us from outer world responsibilities for a time. In my work with depressed and otherwise fatigued individuals, I have found that submission to rest can result in a deeper connection with the dream world. To rest, perchance to dream. This kind of rest, this waking sleep, opens us to the waking dream, that important daytime analogue to the night dream, which we will explore in chapter 9.

Dream Deprivation and Cancer

Although the relationship is complex and inconclusive, scientists have long been interested in links between depression and cancer. Emerging evidence suggests that dream deprivation may also be an important factor in understanding cancer, opening a new avenue of possibilities.

Almost a century ago, Carl Jung and his students began a fascinating exploration of the relationship between depression, dreams, and cancer. Jung believed that cancer was a disease of "extreme extraversion" associated with the loss of one's inner life. I believe that excessive light at night is a significant, overlooked force that encourages extraversion while inhibiting a balanced introversion. With diminished attention to our inner lives, we inevitably deny and repress emotional energies and dreams. Jungians hypothesized that under certain conditions this repressed material is eventually diverted into somatic channels, sometimes manifesting as cancer. Evidence supporting this perspective has been growing ever since.

In 1926, Jung's student Elida Evans published *A Psychological Study of Cancer*, a book investigating cancer risk and personality in which she examined the connection between cancer and schizophrenia. By the nature of their illness, paranoid schizophrenics have a very rich, if out of control, hallucinatory inner life. Hallucinations, which can be understood as an intrusion of dreamlike experiences into waking consciousness, may represent the polar opposite of dream suppression—a kind of dream expulsion. Evans pointed out that paranoid schizophrenics have a strikingly lower incidence of cancer than people without this disorder.

More recent studies confirm that despite the fact that 75 percent to 90 percent of schizophrenics smoke tobacco, they have a significantly lower than average chance of getting lung cancer. Jungians believe that cancer and schizophrenia are opposite expressions of the same essential underlying energies. Schizophrenics express these energies psychologically, through an uncontained and out of control process, while cancer patients do so somatically, silently through their biology and their bodies. Not surprisingly, as a group, schizophrenics are virtually free of fatigue. Could it be that some cancers are a somatic expression of repressed psychological energies?

If dream deprivation is associated with increased cancer risk, will promoting dreaming help us heal? Many contemporary spiritual healers are in agreement with old world shamans about this possibility. There is growing evidence that addresses this question from both psychospiritual as well as biomedical perspectives. As a recent example, Marc Barasch pioneered a fascinating exploration of the role of dreams in healing cancer. Built upon Jungian and spiritual foundations, his book *Healing Dreams: Exploring the Dreams That Can Transform Your Life* (2000) details his personal healing journey from thyroid cancer through dream work.

A number of studies as well as significant anecdotal information suggest that melatonin increases REM sleep. Melatonin has also been shown to decrease the latency of REM periods and is believed to increase sleepiness by relaxing our muscles, taking us a step closer, perhaps, to sleep paralysis. Melatonin levels normally reach their peak in the second half of the night, during the time of our greatest dream activity. Public surveys have shown that melatonin significantly increases the subjective vividness and frequency of dreams as well as dream recall. Given our common resistance to dreaming, it is not surprising that the most common complaint the U.S. Food and Drug Administration receives from melatonin users is that it causes them to dream "too much."

Since melatonin increases dreaming, might it be useful in treating cancer? There is, in fact, a growing body of scientific literature that supports this notion. In a recent series of remarkable animal studies, David E. Blask, Senior Research Scientist at the Bassett Research Institute, has shown melatonin to be remarkably effective in slowing and even stopping tumor growth (2003). For humans, melatonin has been shown to be effective in slowing the growth of a number of nonimmune system cancers. At the University of Arizona's Program in Integrative Medicine we frequently recommend melatonin as an adjunct to cancer treatment. In conjunction with this, I usually encourage cancer patients to make dream work a critical part of their treatment program.

When we are deprived of our dreams, our world flattens and its hues fade. How do we free the black stallion in each of our hearts? In the end, we must develop a deeper regard not only for our dreams but also for the process of dreaming and, perhaps most importantly, for the dreamer residing in each of us.

Regarding Dreams

We disregard our dreams because we consider them weird and intense, but mostly because they threaten our fundamental view of waking reality. In dreams we become free of the constraints that define the waking world—space, time, events—all things are rendered malleable. Dreams violate our gold standard for what is possible. We can experience unimaginable liberation in our dreams as well as the depths of despair. In many respects, dreams are just like waking except much more so.

I believe that most of us intuitively sense that we cannot give our dreams serious attention without it significantly altering our worldviews. Dreams draw us deeply inward. They threaten our extraversion, our blind overcommitment to the outer world and devotion to relentless drive.

Restoring dreams to their rightful place in our lives means we must first guard against dream thieves: the inappropriate use of dream-suppressive substances and medications, and the common dream-dismissive posture of our world. Ultimately, we regard our dreams by simply attending to them, both the big ones and the little ones. Marie ordinarily dismissed her dreams, but given the bigness of her black stallion nightmare, she felt coerced to attend to it. Unfortunately, as the immediacy of her dream faded, so did her resolve to honor the insight it offered. Developing a healthy regard for dreams requires that we develop an intentional and sustained relationship with them. Occasional flirtation gets us nowhere.

Attending to our dreams encourages them to open and reveal their deeper meanings. "A dream unexamined," says the Talmud, "is like a letter unopened." There is a common, virtually universal belief that dreams have meaning—usually latent meaning that must be carefully examined. If we do not consciously select our approach to dreams, we will reflexively approach them in the same way we do our waking lives. There is a common assumption of homogeneity between waking and dreaming that depersonalizes our dreams, shrinking them down to fit more neatly into waking world presumptions. This is what Marie instinctively did when she first interpreted her dream using a dictionary approach.

Marie initially observed her dream through the lens of her waking self or ego, the smaller window through which we view the ordinary waking world. From this perspective, the "I" figure in her dream, the image of Marie sitting in the barn, was synonymous with the "I" figure in her waking life. And everything happening outside of this "I" figure in the dream, then, was not about the dreamer; it was impersonal, just happening to her. This common perspective objectifies and depersonalizes most of the contents of our dreams. By dissociating us from the content of the dream, it also protects us from our own challenging emotions. It downsizes and sanitizes our dreams.

Marie was able to reclaim her dissociated dream content and its related emotion by simply giving a voice to the image of the black stallion. And it spoke. Animals, other people, plants, houses, objects, and essentially anything will speak to us from a dream if we lend it a voice. When dream images speak, all we need to do is listen without preconceptions, judgment, or interpretation.

I generally do not recommend that we "interpret" our dreams in the common understanding of that word. Interpretation is about determining the latent meaning of a dream by analyzing its content in terms of preconceived, waking-world notions. Unless we are doing so as an academic exercise, we generally do not interpret music, art, sunsets, or poetry. We simply attend to and experience them on their own terms to understand their inherent meaning.

Such experience is not derived from an astute, painstaking analytic process but more from a simple kind of de-analysis. In the end, the meaning of a dream simply emerges as we strip away layers of judgments—old encrusted beliefs derived from a lifetime of analysis. Understanding dreams ultimately involves a kind of deconstruction of our initial reactions so that we might meet them on their own terms. We need not construct meaning, only allow it to reveal itself—like an archeological dig where we carefully brush away layers of accretions to expose what was already there and is self-evident.

When Marie finally acknowledged her identification with the stallion, interpretation was unnecessary. Her initial analysis suggesting that the horse was a danger and a bad omen quickly dissipated as a deeper, self-evident truth emerged. She came to realize that this animal's entrapment, its anger, and its desire to be free all belonged to her.

The Talmud goes on to suggest that every dream can have at least twenty-four different meanings. I do not believe this is intended to encourage an exhaustive and obsessive search for every bit of meaning concealed in every dream. Instead, I think it is meant to remind us that dreams come from a very different world than the one we spend most of our waking hours in, a world where simultaneous, multiple levels of meaning reverberate beyond our comprehension.

Just as a thought is the outcome of the underlying process of thinking, a dream is an expression of the underlying process of dreaming. The spiritually fatal flaw in our common approach to dreams is the assumption that we can come to understand them without understanding the place they come from—the world of dreaming. In the end, I believe that even more important than understanding the meaning of any particular dream is coming to know in our hearts that the process of dreaming itself is meaningful.

Regarding Dreaming

As we move from the question, *What might this dream mean?* to the larger concern, *What does dreaming mean?* we venture beyond psychological views of dreaming to encounter a rich variety of spiritual perspectives. We move from the personal to the transpersonal. Contemporary neuroscience and most psychological theories suggest that dreaming is a local phenomenon, a strictly mental or biological process happening here—in this world. In sharp contrast, mystical and spiritual perspectives of dreaming suggest that dreams do not necessarily come from here. They come from some other place.

Dreaming is another world. We are definitely not in Kansas anymore. Cultures and spiritual traditions that revere dreaming recognize that it entails a connection with an alternate reality, another place, another kind of time, another consciousness. There is talk of dreamtime, the dream body, the dreamscape, the dream world. In Western thinking certain kinds of dreams are associated with visits to and from the heavens, the astral planes, other spheres.

Dreaming is to waking as the atmosphere is to the earth. It is made of the same stuff but much lighter and so much larger. Like the atmosphere, dreaming offers us essential containment and spiritual life support. Dreaming is a poetic cushion against our sharply literal lives. It is the spiritual analogue of life in the material world. Dreaming is psychological context, the bigger picture, a subliminal reality. Because we are disconnected from sensory input, dreaming is literally extrasensory perception. And because voluntary movement is inhibited during dreaming, we cannot express ourselves through our bodies. We become disembodied, spirits.

Freud believed dreaming was the "royal road to the unconscious." I believe it is more accurately described as the actual territory. It is the place from which waking consciousness emerges. It is, spiritually speaking, more substantial. "Dreams are not unconscious or subconscious," says my big dreamer friend Susan Pack, "they are superconscious."

Like the horizon, the boundary between the earth and the atmosphere, the line that separates the waking and dreaming world usually appears to be sharp and distinct. But it is not. Billions of tons of earthly matter are swept up into the atmosphere in the form of flying things, dust, and clouds. Likewise, the atmosphere quietly seeps down into the earth, dissolving into the oceans, aerating the crust, and breathing itself into all material life forms. Despite appearances, the horizon is a highly permeable membrane. And so it is with the line between waking and dreaming.

Tibetan Buddhist dream yoga distinguishes *ordinary dreams* from *spiritual dreams*. When the matter of this world is whisked upward into the dream world, it forms our most common, ordinary dreams, those of daily life, work, family, acquaintances, and mundane challenges. Although ordinary dreams are most readily understood in terms of the waking reality they reflect, they occur in the nonordinary atmosphere of the dream world. This new context allows us to see ordinary waking in a nonordinary way.

As the rarefied ethers of the upper atmosphere descend toward the world of matter, they manifest as spiritual dreams. Celestial elements crystallize and settle like snow, like manna, casting a delicate glow around everything. Heaven on Earth. Spiritual dreams are gracious gifts that offer teachings and healings.

Whether they are ordinary, spiritual, or some mix of the two, dreams are born of this other, overarching world. Despite this, we typically approach our dreams as if they were primarily local phenomena—as if they came from this very waking reality or originated strictly in our heads.

Traditional Western spirituality views the waking world as an expression and extension of a larger, spiritual world. *As it is above, so is it below* is a basic Judeo-Christian tenet. It reminds us that Earth was created in the image of heaven. And that we are created in the image of God. When it comes to dreaming, however, we turn this critical spiritual tenet on its head. Just as we tend to depersonalize our dreams, we also de-transpersonalize them. Our approach to dreaming would suggest that the spiritual world is an expression and extension of a more immediate and relevant waking world. As it is below, so is it above.

Rather than receive dreaming as an expression of heaven on Earth, we are dangerously predisposed to projecting the characteristics of Earth onto heaven. This is the same kind of thinking that gives us a God who looks like an old king and angels with bird wings. It constrains our spirituality by sanitizing and downsizing consciousness. And it damages our view of ourselves as dreamers.

Regarding Dreamers

In addition to ordinary and spiritual dreams, Tibetan dream yoga also acknowledges a third, less common kind of dream, the *lucid dream.*

Not long ago I dreamed that I was standing at my bathroom mirror shaving. My hand slipped, and I accidentally lobbed off a substantial chunk of the right wing of my moustache. (Only devout men of facial hair can truly understand how bad this felt.) I was shocked, saddened, and perplexed. Faced with the difficult challenge of what to do, I carefully considered my options. Since I had had a moustache for my entire adult life, I was ambivalent about shaving it off completely. I also quickly dismissed thoughts about trimming the left side to match the right. Too much a retro, Errol Flynn look. As I continued to stare hard into the mirror of my dream, studying this reflection of myself, it occurred to me that I had another option. I could simply let it be. "Since I'm dreaming," I thought, "my original moustache will be back when I awaken in the morning." I felt quite relieved.

We have seen that we cannot fully appreciate the meaning of dreams without exploring the meaning of dreaming. Likewise, to better understand dreaming, we need to consider the dreamer. Obviously, the dreamer, the part of us doing the dreaming, is present, whether accounted for or not, in all dreams. At the opening of this chapter I suggested that when we dream, we usually believe we are awake. The dreamer is present in these dreams but not accounted for until actually awakening. My moustache dream illustrates lucid dreaming, dreaming where the dreamer is aware of dreaming during the dream, accounted for prior to awakening.

"Our truest life is when we are in dreams awake," said Henry David Thoreau. Lucid dreaming has been a topic of great psychological and spiritual interest for centuries. In recent years, scientific studies have confirmed this phenomenon. Lucidity in dreams is probably more common than we believe. Many people experience a partial awakening during a dream, usually a bad dream or nightmare. A faint awareness arises that they are, in fact, in bed, asleep, and dreaming. And even though awakening fully might bring some relief, people frequently choose to remain in their dream to see how it will finish. You might recall that Marie reported some spontaneous lucidity as her nightmare was ending: ". . . I start to feel myself gradually waking up. Part of me is so relieved as I begin to realize I'm sleeping and it's just a dream. But, it's strange; part of me still wants to see what the horse will do."

The essence of lucidity is not, as many people believe, about the ability to control one's dreams. The common Western inclination to impose control on lucid dreams can distract us from their deeper value and meaning. In contrast, Tibetan dream yoga encourages gradually withdrawing attention from the contents of the dream and focusing more on the dreamer. The essence of lucidity is not about control but about recognizing the important role of the dreamer in the dreaming process. The more we recognize ourselves as dreamers, the better we can come to understand how the mind creates not only dreams but also the waking dream and what we consider waking reality.

When God chose to create Eve, He caused a deep sleep, or *tardema*, in the old Hebrew, to fall upon Adam. Tardema is interpreted variously as a deep sleep, what we might understand as an altered state of consciousness or even a spiritual dream state. In Modern Hebrew, the term *tardema* is associated with general anesthesia. This seems fitting given that Adam was about to have one of his ribs removed, presumably a painful experience. "And Adam slept," says the Old Testament.

Author and spiritual pioneer Hugh Prather points out that nowhere in the remainder of Genesis, even long after the creation of Eve, are we advised that Adam was awakened. Was this a divine oversight? Perhaps a lengthy recovery is to be expected following the surgical separation of the genders. Or, is Adam still asleep? Could it be that all subsequent creation is merely the dream of Adam?

The notion that life is but a dream is one of the most universal spiritual teachings. It reminds us of the ultimate transpersonal nature of the dreamer. Whether it is maya in Hinduism, illusion in Buddhism, or the dream in Western traditions, this theme echoes persistently throughout spiritual teachings across time and around the world.

The recognition that we are dreaming is critical to our spiritual awakening. By definition, we know that we will eventually awaken from a dream. In lucid dreaming we become aware that we are in a dream not by becoming aware of the dream but by becoming aware of ourselves as dreamers. Because it offers certain knowledge of a pending awakening, realizing that one is a dreamer can render even the darkest nightmares tolerable. Likewise, cultivating and deepening our awareness that life is but a dream—that waking itself is a kind of dreaming—opens the way for an even greater awakening.

In *Parables from Other Planets,* Hugh and Gayle Prather beautifully illustrate the essential truth about dreams, dreaming, and dreamers:

> The town of Vaduz is nestled within the Great Bridge that spans the binary planets of Orb and Bex. This natural land bridge or Fusion supports the numerous thoroughfares connecting the planets, and the most popular vehicle is very similar to the automobiles seen on Earth, with an added air-cushion generator that allows the cars to plane at higher velocities.
>
> There was once a mother living in Vaduz who discovered that she could enter her son's dreams at will. One night the child began thrashing in his sleep. Instantly the mother saw that her son was in a driverless car that was speeding out of control. She closed her eyes and started to enter his dream, but suddenly she stopped. Many times before she had made the changes in his dreams that she had thought he would want, but the dreams had always turned again to discord. She knew that she had the ability to apply the brake and stop the car, but being wiser now she saw that a disturbed dream is caused by a disturbed dreamer, and no matter how it is altered, it cannot reflect more peace than the dreamer himself possesses. Wanting now only to bring peace to his mind, she lifted her son up. In the dream, the car flew off the road and started falling. She held her son securely in her arms. In the dream he saw the walls of the car closing in. She sang a lullaby of her love and of her son's eternal safety. In the dream he saw the choir start to sing at his own funeral. Yet slowly the child began to feel the warm presence of his mother enfolding him, and as he awoke to the reality of her love, his dream ended. (1991, 3–4)

Healing Dream Practices

The following practices are offered to assist in developing a more personal relationship with your dreams, the world of dreaming, and yourself as a dreamer.

Guard against Dream Thieves

Given the prevalence of dream deprivation in our world today, it is important to be cognizant of dream thieves. Anything that disrupts our sleep can disrupt dreaming. The desire to maintain a healthy dream life becomes another reason to make healthy sleep a priority.

I have emphasized that many sleep and antidepressant medications disrupt REM sleep. If you are taking any of these, check with your physician or pharmacist to determine if your medication may in fact be disrupting your dreams. Consider other options and alternatives with your doctor. Remember that alcohol also interferes with REM sleep. Women need to be particularly cautious about evening alcohol consumption since they generally are able to tolerate only about half the amount of alcohol that men can.

Open to Dream Life

Many people report difficulties with recalling their dreams. This can usually be remedied with the proper intent and practice. Set an intention to dream and to remember your dreams. We remember dreams in much the same way we remember waking experiences, by paying attention to them. Begin to conscientiously attend to dreams and dreaming. Think, talk, write, and read about them.

Resume the last position you were asleep in upon awakening. Without searching for dreams, become mindful of any emotions you have, allowing yourself to feel them. When dream images begin to arise, do not pursue them; allow them to come to you. Make note of even faint or isolated images. If no dreams or dream images arise, make note of whatever emotions you notice.

Consider the possibility that there is no such thing as a bad dream. Certainly there are dreams that are uncomfortable, disconcerting, and nightmarish. When we discuss shadow, we will see that there are positive elements concealed in even the most unsettling dreams. We can practice courage by planning to face any and all adversity in our dreams. We cannot be hurt by our dreams. It is not true that if you die in your dream, for example, you will die in reality. Keep in mind that dreams cannot harm you even though they may stir up very strong emotion.

Record Your Dreams

Consider keeping a written account of your dream experiences in a journal. Make note of dreams, dream images, and any other related associations that may accompany them. It is best to do this upon arising, since our recollection will tend to fade as the day proceeds.

Reviewing one's dream journal entries periodically can reveal interesting themes and patterns in your dream life. Dream journaling can be integrated with a daily diary as well as a waking dream journal, which we will discuss in chapter 9. If you are drawn to actively interpret your dreams, avoid rigid dictionary approaches. Instead, consider more open-ended gestalt dream therapy or archetypal psychology approaches.

Establish Dream Communities

One of the most effective ways of deepening our relationship with the dream world is to address dreams in community. Routinely sharing dreams with a spouse or partner as we arise in the morning is an effective way to deepen intimacy. Once again, there is no need for "analysis." Simply listen and share your thoughts and feelings about the dream experience and imagery. Think of this as if you had been on separate journeys overnight and have come together to share your stories.

Dreams can also become part of morning sharing in families. Many cultures around the world ritually share dreams in the morning. In the same way we might ask children how their days went at school, we can establish a routine of asking them about how their nights went in the dream world.

Consider sharing dreams on a regular basis with close friends as well. A recent dream can be intentionally woven into a catch-up conversation over lunch. When we include dreams as a part of the discussion of other meaningful life experiences, we lend a deeper sense of credence to them.

Dreams can be brought into community in a more formal way through establishing dream circles. Dream circles refer to regular, ongoing small-group meetings that offer a safe and supportive forum for sharing and discussing dreams and dreaming. Morning or breakfast dream circles have the advantage of being more closely positioned to our dream lives.

~

Dreaming is the internal representation of early morning, a kind of spiritual gestation period preceding our rebirth into the waking world. We dream primarily under the auspices of the night sky as it resolves slowly back into day, as the atmosphere reconstitutes with light and form. I believe that opening one's heart and mind to the dream world is a courageous and irrevocable act. When we push past our fear and judgment and dare to go to the edge, we witness a vast and infinite expanse beyond our wildest imagination. We can never be complacent with living in the box of mundanity again. Opening to the dream world changes the way we look at life and ourselves forever, and we will not want to go back.

~6

Dawn: A Gradual Awakening

The breeze at dawn has secrets to tell you; don't go back to sleep.
You must ask for what you really want; don't go back to sleep.
People are going back and forth across the doorsill
where the two worlds meet.
The door is round and open; don't go back to sleep.

—RUMI

I HAVE A DISTINCT MEMORY of gradual morning awakenings as a young boy on our family's farm in South Jersey. Even from deep within my dreams I could sense fresh light trickling into my bedroom and hear sparrows chirping. These were permeable dreams, inviting dawn's gentle glow and bird songs into their story lines. The night world of sleep and dreams melded seamlessly with the new day's waking. Like the advent of dawn, waking was patient and peaceful. It was a new day, and although still unnamed, it brimmed with the innocent possibilities of childhood. It was as if I was not awakened by the world but rather awakened with it.

Although somewhat less distinct, I also have memories of awakenings as a teenager. Since I had discovered the music alarm clock, my morning dreams were no longer infused with the songs of birds but with those of the Byrds, the Beatles, and other rockers. Life in the city and culture was now considerably more interesting to me than nature. And the anxious demands of adolescence quickly trumped the remnants of my vivid dreams. While shielding my eyes from the morning light with a pillow, I quickly calculated what day it was. I could already smell the donuts from the bakery across the street as I wondered what to wear to school that day.

And then there are the memories of awakenings from my young adult years—many that I would rather forget. My bedroom was now positioned to minimize that harsh morning sun, which always seemed to rise too soon. But it could not block out the rumble of suburbia rousing itself like a monster recovering from a bad blow. Then came the jolting shrill of my alarm, the slap of the snooze button, and the nagging of my bladder. I found myself in routine conflict between abject grogginess and the reveille call echoing in my head: *It's getting late!* It always was. *What? Is that the garbage truck? Oh, crap—it's only Tuesday?* The newspaper thumped at the front door. A world of events beckoned as my to-do list began chirping annoyingly in the background. Finally, the aromatic lure of my automatic coffee pulled me over the top. I hardly ever remembered my dreams. And I rarely felt as if I got enough sleep.

Given its powerful influence on the quality of our days, morning awakening is a surprisingly neglected topic. From a sleep science perspective, waking up is about negotiating a quick and tricky biological transition from sleep to the waking state. In mechanical terms, we are rapidly rebooted or switched back on. In sharp contrast, however, sacred traditions around the world encourage a more measured, prayerful, and mindful approach to morning.

More so than about falling asleep, we do seem to have an intuitive sense that awakening is a process—a gradual process. If prematurely roused, we are apt to say, "I'm not awake yet," or "I'm still sleeping," suggesting at least some awareness that we do not awaken in a flash. Exploring morning awakening as a gradual process reveals that it is a rich and complex phase of consciousness characterized by unique possibility—as well as heightened vulnerability.

Heart attacks and certain kinds of strokes are most common around awakening, most asthma attacks occur between 4:00 a.m. and 7:00 a.m., migraines are most likely to occur in the morning, and most hospital deaths occur near dawn. Of less interest to science, anecdotal reports suggest that creative and artistic inspiration is most readily accessed in the morning. Big dreams seem especially abundant as we transition to awakening. And sacred epiphanies seem to occur more frequently with sunrise meditations.

Why is morning awakening a time of such vulnerability and possibility? To borrow a mechanistic metaphor, we are shifting gears, turning a corner. We are driving over those bumpy tracks that divide the relatively safe neighborhood of night, sleep, and dreams from the more challenging region of day and waking.

Awakening can be best understood in terms of a complex body-mind process, associated with crucial biological and psychological changes. It is indeed darkest before the dawn. Like the outer world, it is cool and "dark" inside of us as we are coming to. Our dream-sustaining melatonin levels have peaked as our core body temperature simultaneously reached its nadir. We are deeply internal at this time, normally immersed in our most protracted period of dreaming. With our voluntary muscles off-line, the body is heavy with sleep paralysis—in a state of cool suspension.

Awakening normally involves a complex cascade of biological and psychological changes that carry the mind from dreaming to waking and the body from suspension to activity. As Nyx descends from the night sky, we experience an analogous drop in melatonin, a steady increase in body temperature, and a resurgence of cortisol. As the sun rises to illuminate and energize the hemisphere, so do our cortisol levels rise to energize us. (It is time we get past the bad rap that attempts to reduce cortisol to a "stress hormone" and acknowledge that it plays a critical and positive role in the mediation of energy.) With these changes, we are carried from the world of dreams, thawed from our biological suspension, and prepared for reentry into the waking world.

Like dawn, awakening is simultaneously a time of night and day, and, paradoxically, a time of neither night nor day. As the mind transits from dreaming to waking, it passes through a hybrid zone of consciousness known as the *hypnopompic state*. Hypnopompic suggests a movement away from sleep. It is characterized by a kind of fuzzy awareness, as if one eye is fluttering to peer out at the world, while the other remains closed and turned inward. In this half-wake, half-dream state our attention is shifting from the dream world but is not yet oriented to the waking world.

Likewise, as the body progresses from dream suspension to waking activity, it also crosses a hybrid zone of biology. Although we might sense our waking energies gradually returning, we are still heavy with the residual fatigue of sleep paralysis. The body is naturally languid in the hypnopompic state.

By nature, awakening is much like a birth. It delivers us, disoriented and languid, through a narrow passage from one world to another world. It invites us to begin sensing and moving, but ever so slowly. A gradual awakening carries us through a lush coastal zone of consciousness that holds immense personal potential. Misunderstood, disregarded, and even disparaged in common culture, this exceptional experience is commonly referred to as grogginess. Derived circuitously from an English rum drink, grogginess is a certain cue for most of us to snap out of it—to intentionally hasten our awakening.

If we wish to explore the spiritual possibilities of awakening in earnest, we must begin by considering that the morning grogginess we routinely seek to dismiss may be well worth exploring. *The breeze at dawn has secrets to tell you,* says Rumi. Lingering in bed for a few extra moments upon awakening does not mean we are lazy or depressed.

For many, morning awakenings are among the most mindless of experiences. We pay about as much attention to our personal experience of arising each day as we do to the sunrise. Why should we? Most of us awaken badly, unrefreshed, with bothersome bladders, bad breath, and bed head. When we add the noxious effects of widespread sleep and dream deprivation, hangovers from substance and sleeping pill use, and the time pressures of modern industrial life to the mix, we have a formula for another kind of common morning sickness.

Too many of us awaken in a manner similar to the way we were born. It is less a natural childbirth, more of a forceps delivery. Or a caesarian section. Less an emergence and more an emergency. If the process of awakening is the birth of our day, then morning is its early childhood, a critical developmental phase in the life of each new day. How we awaken, how we posture toward morning establishes a powerful psychospiritual trajectory for the remainder of the day. We can ignite and launch ourselves like a rocket ship—a rude awakening. Or, inspired by dawn's new light, we can blossom, fresh, wet, and vibrant with sacred possibility—a good morning.

Rude Awakenings

Our natural grogginess, this proclivity to arise gradually, languid and disoriented, is lost in the scamper to start the day. Under pressure to quickly reorient, reenergize, and resume our incessant drive, we have no time for slow starts.

A majority of Americans awaken unsatisfied, underslept, and exhausted from chronic and mounting sleep debt. Others, having knocked themselves out the night before with alcohol, pot, or sleeping pills, must now pay the piper. It is as if we awaken in need of emergency cognitive defibrillation to counter our sleep-deprived or substance-aggravated grogginess. We can manage to awaken only with the aid of alarms, an infusion of counterfeit energy, and a jolt of hyperbolic morning news.

Too many people have firsthand experience with morning-after hangovers following excessive evening alcohol or drug indulgence. Most are probably not aware of the dampening effects that even moderate use of such substances can have on our morning. And many others are completely unaware of the subtle and sometimes extensive drowsiness associated with their sleeping pill use.

In sharp contrast to sleeping pill ads depicting images of impossibly perky morning-after awakenings, most sleeping pills damage our morning consciousness. Despite its clever name, Ambien, the most popular prescription sleeping pill in the world today, does not truly deliver on the promise of a good (bien) morning (am). In fact, extensive research on sleeping pills, including the over-the-counter varieties, suggests that they commonly result in morning-after cognitive deficits. In this way, sleeping pills can complicate our natural morning disorientation.

The notion of a gradual awakening flies in the face of expectations that we start up like a machine. It makes sense that in a mechanistic world so many of us are awakened abruptly by an electric alarm clock. According to the National Sleep Foundation (2004), more than one-half of all American adults say they need an alarm clock to get up in the morning. Nearly 70 percent of young adults ranging from eighteen to twenty-nine years cannot awaken without an alarm. By definition, an alarm—as in a fire or a burglar alarm—signals danger. Too often we ignite the day with a spark of fear and stress. A shot of adrenaline is fired, the gates open. In response, millions will slap their snooze buttons.

For many of us, the screech of the alarm clock signals the unofficial start of morning rush hour. During our stolen snooze, we remain semiconscious that the race has started; the countdown for launching of the day is already under way. We have a designated number of minutes to get prepared, suited up, and refueled for takeoff. And this is all the more challenging if we also have a crew of children or other family members to launch.

When we finally manage to drag ourselves out of bed, we grope for an antidote to our lethargy—for quick energy. We seek our usual fuel: refined sugary foods and, of course, caffeine, most usually in the form of coffee. We wake up and smell the coffee. Or is it the other way around? Just the thought of coffee beckons millions of bleary-eyed people out of bed. According to the National Coffee Association (2000), coffee fumes ignite the engines of over 100 million of us every day. And as we begin to sufficiently rouse our languid bodies, we become energized enough to address our disorientation.

We most commonly reorient to the new day by obtaining information. Even before getting out of bed most of us have instinctively oriented to time—not just the hour but also the day of the week. As we will see, the knowledge of when it is provides fundamental definition to our day. After arising there is a natural inclination to assess what is new in the waking world we had left behind. For the majority of us, this is not about the world of nature, a sunrise, the weather, or a fresh blossom, but about the world of culture, politics, economics, and human drama and tragedy. Most of us reorient not through the newness of morning but through the morning news. Millions of Americans routinely access morning news within moments of arising, through television, newspapers, radio, and the Internet. Such news provides us with navigational coordinates to guide our morning launch into the new day's trajectory. A common fantasy of a really good morning—lingering in bed with a cup of coffee and the *Times*.

Rude awakenings are less about awakening, more about igniting our engines and launching into the day like a rocket. We are machines that refuel with caffeine and navigate with news. We awaken through preparatory activities with little or no regard for the night we are leaving. Like sleepy crud in our eyes, night is seen as a film of grogginess that clouds our consciousness—something that needs to be sanitized, wiped away before we can start our day.

A Good Morning

How else might we awaken? Henry David Thoreau offers another view in *Walden*:

> I love a broad margin to my life. Sometimes in a
> summer morning . . . I sat in my sunny doorway
> from sunrise to noon, rapt in reverie, amidst the
> pines and hickories and sumacs in undisturbed soli-
> tude and stillness. . . . I grew in those seasons like
> corn in the night, and they were far better than any
> work of the hands would have been. (1854, 85)

For a few luckier souls, morning awakening is a slow and gentle process characterized by lingering in that limbic zone between dreaming and waking. Even if we do not take a margin as broad as Thoreau's, a good morning finds us patient with, and even enjoying, our low energy as well as our lack of orientation to the day. We are aware of and happy to explore our grogginess. A good morning offers a gradual awakening, naturally inspired and energized by the sunrise—inside and out. Awakening becomes a warm celebration of an unbranded newness that redefines everything. A good morning is informed by a deeply refreshed sense of mystery.

If we can get past our initial judgment that our grogginess is dull and meaningless, it emerges as a secret portal to this mystery. It is a lush coastal region of extraordinary experience, a sacred morning fog through which we can witness our ordinary sense of self gradually reemerging, remaking itself. Because we are not really half-asleep when groggy, but half-dreaming, it is also a channel for remarkable creative expression, a place to find new ideas, inspiration, and healing.

When was the last time we came up with the sun instead of an alarm? As the most obvious defining characteristic of morning, the advent of light is the primary source of energy for our planet. Sunrise warms the earth, awakening and energizing all living things. And like an internal sun, our biological fires also steadily rise in the morning. If we are patient with morning, we learn that we need not depend on caffeine and news to wake and orient us. The sun does not rise with the flip of a switch. Neither should we expect to.

A good morning gradually reorients us through newness. It casts a fresh light on everything and everyone emerging from night. Although most things may appear unchanged, we sense that they have been subtly remade by the night. And we are new as well. Our sense of self, which had dissolved into sleep and dreams, is now reconstituting. We awaken remade, reconfigured, and innocent. In *Women Who Run with the Wolves*, Clarissa Pinkola Estes describes this process as reflected in myth:

> If you could lay your eyes upon the most fire-hardened, most cruel and pitying person alive . . . at the moment of waking you would see in them for a moment the untainted child spirit, the pure innocent. In sleep we are once again brought back to a state of sweetness. In sleep we are remade. We are

reassembled from the inside out, fresh and new as
innocents. (1992, 151)

A good morning offers a unique vantage. Through a gradual
awakening as innocents, we see the world and ourselves anew. It
is a nonjudgmental kind of perception with qualities reminiscent
of the dream. Our natural morning grogginess is, in fact, our first
waking dream. It is a permeable passageway in which the inner
world of dreaming and the outer world of waking cannot yet be
segregated. Here, we can witness our own rebirth into the new day.
A good morning reorients us with our own sacred newness.

It is not surprising to find a preponderance of morning meditation, prayer, and ritual throughout spiritual and religious traditions. Reflecting an archetypal recognition of the wondrous possibilities inherent in dawn, morning spiritual practices have an
intentional slowness. Such practices would certainly fly in the face
of our incessant drive. I believe that morning prayer, meditation,
and ritual, particularly if personalized, are a natural expression of
a good morning.

Lucid Awakening

The breeze at dawn has secrets to tell you.

In contrast to petitionary prayer, which is essentially a statement
of what we want, contemplative prayer emphasizes listening. A
gradual awakening begins with our listening to what morning is
saying to us.

Since awakening is the internal representation of dawn, we can
listen to the sunrise as well as to our own rising. Attending to the
breeze at dawn, to the gentle advent of light, both literally and
figuratively, teaches us about the process of illumination. Unlike
day, in which things are lit up, awakening is about the alchemical
transformation of darkness into light. As we will see in chapter 8,
this process is crucial in shadow work. It is also fundamental to

the Western creation myth. The very creation of the universe as depicted in the Old Testament emphasizes the emergence of light from darkness.

In practicing lucid awakening, we become privy to the secrets of creation.

You must ask for what you really want.

It is only after listening that we are better able to speak our truth. With a deepening understanding of the essence of creation, we are better able to ask for what we really want. We are able to set a conscious trajectory, to intentionally reorient to the new day.

It is interesting to note how much effort most of us invest in setting a conscious trajectory for the physical aspects of our days. We take great care in preparing our bodies, our homes, our autos, and our workplaces for the day. We must also be willing to nurture our minds and spirits through intentional orientation to the day.

Intentional orientation may be the most common theme of morning prayers across traditions. Morning prayers and rituals are about setting deliberate spiritual trajectories for our day as we arise into it. Prayer and ritual not only establish a direction—a conscious realignment with values we want to live by—but as importantly, they set a tempo, a pace for the day. They establish our rhythm.

In helping us align with our deepest intention, morning prayer and ritual protect us from being swept away by the high tide of industrial culture. If we fail to orient consciously through personal intention, we will keep orienting unconsciously through cultural convention.

People are going back and forth across the doorsill where the two worlds meet.

Dawn is a dimly lit but highly permeable passageway between night and day. Awakening, then, can be seen less as a relinquishment of night and more as an integration of night into day. Like mushrooms that germinate overnight, we can carry the sustenance of the darkness with us into the day. Awakening need not be based on the dismissal of sleep and dream experiences; it can just as well build on and integrate them. Can we allow ourselves to open simultaneously to elements of both, of darkness and light, of night and day, and of dreaming and waking? In doing so, we practice the challenging task of balancing our awareness between the inner and outer worlds, between fundamental aspects of duality.

Both Eastern and Western religions associate morning with sacred rebirth. Just as Tibetan Buddhism views sleep onset as a spiritual form of dying, it views morning awakening as synonymous with birth. Likewise, the resurrection of Christ is said to have occurred in the morning and has been associated with the sacred promise of a new day. The term *resurrection* is derived from the notion of resurgence—a coming back again. Morning is the resurrection of waking life.

The door is round and open.

As we begin to awaken, we encounter the question, *where am I?*— the common experience of orienting to place. There is the deeper question, *when am I?* (or when is it?)—the somewhat less conscious experience of orienting to time. And then there is the most fundamental question, usually outside of our awareness, *who am I?*—the question that orients us to our known, named selves. Our responses, whether conscious and intentional or unconscious and reflexive, orient us to time, place, and person.

I was not surprised to realize that these three questions form the framework for a basic psychiatric screening known as the mental status exam. This quick screening is designed to determine if an individual is essentially in touch with reality. In professional talk, we ask if patients "are oriented 'times three'"—if they are oriented to person, place, and time.

When Am I?

As we gradually regain ordinary waking consciousness, we reorient ourselves to time. We might remember, for example, that it is

Monday and we need to go to work, or that it is Saturday and we can breathe a sigh of relief. Roger Miller said, "Every day is Saturday if you're a dog." Since we are not, the day, month, season, and year (and the meanings associated with these) into which we awaken will have a potent effect on our day's psychological and spiritual trajectory. *When it is* creates a temporal structure that contributes to defining both our behavior and our sense of self.

Where Am I?

On occasion, particularly if we are traveling, we may find ourselves consciously trying to orient to place. Many people have had the experience of awakening away from home and momentarily not remembering where they were. I believe that this orienting to place actually occurs in a subtler, semiconscious manner on a daily basis, even when we are at home. Like orienting to time, where we are, as well as the different meanings associated with various places, can profoundly influence our day and our sense of self.

Who Am I?

Much less obvious during the awakening process is our reorientation to person—to who we are. Anecdotal evidence suggests we can awaken and become at least partially aware even prior to having regained our personal identity. It is as if we have not yet claimed our name.

Perhaps you have had the occasional experience of awakening refreshed and peaceful only to suddenly remember a crisis brewing in your life. We can awaken momentarily to a deeper, more peaceful, prenamed sense of self only to have our worldly identity and personality abruptly downloaded. Although this peaceful sense of self is easily discounted as a kind of groggy forgetfulness, I believe it is actually a spontaneous spiritual remembrance, one that can be intentionally cultivated through the practice of lucid awakening.

Such a practice allows us to develop a relationship with a deeper, perhaps unnamed aspect of self that lives outside of time, place, and personality. Cultivating awareness of the process of awakening encourages an expansion of personal consciousness. It provides a new understanding of how we reconstruct our identities on a daily basis, of how we are reborn.

Don't go back to sleep.

Morning awakening is a time of spiritual opportunity. Permeability between night and day, dreaming and waking, and consciousness and unconsciousness is great at dawn. The practice of lucid awakening can deepen our sense of freedom to choose how and even who we want to be—to choose our rebirth. Can we avoid falling again and again with each new morning back into a kind of sleep we believe to be waking? Can we carry the elements of a new awakening and a sacred morning vision with us into the day?

Morning Light

In his book *Spontaneous Healing,* Dr. Andrew Weil shares a story about Shin-ichiro Terayama, a Japanese friend who experienced a spontaneous, rather miraculous healing from cancer. After struggling with and finally dismissing conventional treatments, Shin, who was gravely ill, decided to use alternative medical approaches and, against medical advice, left the hospital one morning. Dr. Weil writes:

> When Shin awoke the next day, he was amazed
> to find himself alive. The morning seemed to him
> unbearably beautiful, and he was aware of a great
> desire to watch the sun rise. He went to the eighth-
> floor rooftop of his apartment house, where he could
> look over the skyline of Tokyo. He recited Buddhist
> mantras and poems, put his hands together to pray,
> and awaited the sun. When it rose, he felt a ray enter
> his chest, sending energy through his body. "I felt

something wonderful was going to happen, and I
started to cry," he says. "I was just so happy to be
alive. I saw the sun as God."... During the next few
weeks Shin ... performed daily the important ritual
of watching the sun rise from his roof—the one
thing he looked forward to each day. (1995, 102)

Morning light is healing. This is not to suggest that anyone can
replicate Shin's experience or even that it was the light exposure,
per se, that healed Shin. In all likelihood, it was about the interaction of his treatments, the morning light, and Shin's commitment and faith.

Thanks in large part to the field of sleep medicine, the role of
light in health and illness has received growing attention in recent
years. Morning light is the most potent zeitgeber. As discussed in
chapter 2, our personal clock is reset daily by morning light. This
clock regulates the circadian timing of an elaborate symphony of
biological events, playing a key role in maintaining health.

In addition to regulating our circadian rhythms, morning light
influences other complex biological and psychological processes.
Just as dusk signals our need to slow, turn inward, and eventually
sleep, morning light naturally awakens, activates, and draws our
attention outward toward the world. Morning light stimulates the
release of serotonin, a well-known wakefulness neurotransmitter
associated with energy, activation, and focused attention. Specific
wavelengths present in natural morning light also stem melatonin
production, further diminishing our sleepiness.

Why is morning light different from the other daylight? As the
sun heats the earth during daylight hours, convection currents of
warm air stir dust particles into the atmosphere. This dust filters
certain wavelengths out of the natural light spectrum, resulting
in the increased redness we sometimes see at sunset. During the
night, however, the earth cools, allowing this atmospheric dust to
settle to the ground. By morning, the sun rises into a refreshed,
clarified, and receptive sky. First morning light offers a safe, natural,
full-spectrum optical elixir. Because it is indirect and filtered

through more atmosphere, early morning light is also considerably safer than midday light. This first light is the organic, whole-grain equivalent of illumination. It is not surprising that Shin was drawn to greet the dawn as a source of healing and spiritual inspiration.

We have long known that light therapy, or phototherapy, is useful in treating seasonal affective disorder, a kind of depression associated with diminished light exposure through the winter season. In recent years, light therapy has shown significant promise in treating more common forms of clinical depression as well. A number of studies suggest that depressed people may experience a pattern of chronically delayed melatonin offset. We saw earlier that as we approach awakening, our melatonin levels normally begin to drop. When they do not, we awaken into a depressive trajectory, feeling excessively heavy and unable to meet the demands of the new day.

Since morning light curbs melatonin production, it makes sense that it might also diminish symptoms of depression. Recent studies have shown that regular morning light exposure may be at least as effective as standard antidepressant medication in ameliorating clinical depression. This is particularly true if the program of light exposure is initiated following a full or partial night of sleep deprivation. Sleep deprivation is known to temporarily reduce symptoms of depression but has not been widely used as a treatment because symptoms quickly rebound when normal sleeping is resumed. When one full or even partial night of sleep deprivation is coupled with an ongoing regimen of light exposure, the positive effects can more readily be sustained over time. A growing body of research suggests that phototherapy may be the most promising treatment available today for clinical depression. Dr. Daniel Kripke, whose work in opposition to sleeping pills was mentioned earlier, offers free access to a Web-based book titled *Brighten Your Life* (2002), which provides a detailed review of phototherapy.

When natural morning light is not readily accessible due to weather or other limitations, there is the option of using phototherapy devices. "Light boxes," special desk lamps, illuminated visors, and other similar products designed to deliver therapeutic doses of light have been shown to be effective. During the protracted northern winter season, The Café Engel, in Helsinki, Finland, offers its customers a standard menu of continental breakfasts with a free side of a light box.

A Note on Dark Mornings

As wondrous as the possibilities of gradual morning awakenings are, they will not necessarily deter our personal darkness. Virtually all of us have experienced dark mornings. We sometimes awaken from bad dreams, from bad nights, or into bad days. If we do manage to get some sleep during a crisis, temporarily forgetting our struggles, we may feel assaulted anew by the resurgence of pain when we awaken. As much as my mother loved dusk and night, I am certain she struggled with dawn and daylight. Morning does not consistently promise healing, but it does offer a sense of newness, a sense of possibilities. Possibilities will not relieve us of our struggles, but if we are open and receptive to them, they will offer us hope.

Lucid Awakening Practices

Bringing more awareness to the process of morning awakenings can have a positive impact on the quality of your days. The following practices are offered to help you more readily access the promise inherent in dawn.

Lose Your Alarm Clock

Whenever possible, allow yourself to awaken without an alarm. With sufficient sleep you will find it easy to awaken naturally in the morning. If you must use an alarm, as an alternative to the jarring type, consider using a dawn simulator that awakens one slowly with gradually increasing illumination. Notice how differently you come to without an alarm.

Practice Gradual Awakenings

Establish a habit of gradual, lucid morning awakenings. Plan to regularly linger in bed with your eyes closed for a few moments as you are awakening. If you need more time for this, adjust your sleep schedule to allow a margin of a few extra moments when you are arising. Let yourself awaken slowly. Stephen Levine, author of *A Gradual Awakening*, encourages becoming mindful of which breath you awaken with. Is it the in breath or the out breath?

Explore your morning grogginess. Become aware of bodily sensations as well as mental images, observing these without analysis or judgment. Through your grogginess, notice how your mind orients to the day by asking where and when it is. With practice, try to become mindful of your identity as it reemerges from sleep and dreams to the waking state.

Notice the thought that immediately precedes your opening your eyes and getting out of bed. Perhaps a thought about the demands of the day or the nagging of your bladder? These thoughts are the intentions that define our initial movement into the day. Do we arise in reaction to bodily or mental pressures? Can we arise to the lure of a positive, passionate pursuit? Experiment with selecting a conscious intention that will inspire rather than coax you out of bed. Notice the impact on the quality of your morning as well as your day.

As you continue your morning, consider your intentions for the day as a means of setting a conscious morning trajectory—a good morning. Beyond what you would like to happen—any objectives you wish to attain—think about the quality of the day you would like to have. Beyond consideration of what you would like to do, reflect on how you would like to do it, the state of mind you wish to cultivate throughout the day, independent of events.

Keep a journal about your lucid awakening experiences. Notice any connections between your dreams, the quality of your awakening, and the quality of your day. If you have a sleep partner, share your experiences of mindful awakening. If you are able to do so

without disturbing your awareness, gently talk about the process
as it is happening.

Take a Morning Light Bath

Consider establishing a routine of morning light exposure for twenty
or thirty minutes each day. Get outside as soon as you can after arising. You might couple this with a gentle walk or just relax outdoors
in a quiet and comfortable spot. Notice the variable qualities of
morning light, particularly the platinum glow of the sun's corona
just before it breaks the horizon.

Engage in Morning Spiritual Practices

Explore specific morning prayers, meditations, and other practices
associated with your personal religious or spiritual tradition. If you
are not affiliated with any particular tradition, you might enjoy sampling approaches from various Western, Eastern, and indigenous
world traditions. Hugh Prather's *Morning Notes: 365 Meditations to
Wake You Up* offers daily readings to help define a conscious, spiritual trajectory for each new day. Experiment with integrating these
into a personalized morning routine.

Try approaching the seemingly mundane aspects of your morning routine, including cleansing, getting dressed, and your first
meal, in a sacred manner.

Try a Morning News Fast

Consider experimenting with a morning news fast for a number
of days. Try to satisfy your innate quest for morning newness by
exploring more natural changes in yourself and your environment.
Look up at the sky.

~

Rumi's admonishment *don't go back to sleep* is not about the risks of hitting your snooze button. Modern life ushers us much too quickly through the passage of awakening. Such rude awakenings prevent us from catching a glimpse of the sacredness inherent in the new day. Beyond the obvious, enticing metaphor of ultimate spiritual awakening, there is great value in setting a conscious trajectory for our day. We have a choice about how we will come to.

⌁ 7

Waking: The Daze of Our Lives

Man was made at the end of the week's work when God was tired.

—MARK TWAIN

"COFFEE!" MARY WHISPERED with a raspy, plaintive tone as she stretched one hand to turn on the shower while frantically brushing her teeth with the other. She had overslept her alarm. Still sleepy and fatigued, Mary, a thirty-something mother of two teenagers, was swept into the start of another day with a whirlwind of self-rebuke. *Why did I go to bed so late again . . . had to do the bills . . . shouldn't have stayed up watching that dumb film. Oh . . . got to remember to take my Prozac.* She squinted at the watch on the sink. *Damn, it's late! I'll just give the kids some pop tarts. And I need to stop and get gas. And coffee!* she thought again, as she finished her shower. Coffee was her inspiration, her morning prayer.

Insufficient sleep syndrome is the most common sleep disorder in America and probably in the industrialized world. According to the National Sleep Foundation (2005), nearly 75 percent of American adults routinely cut their sleep short, resulting in what appears to be a "voluntary" insomnia. Given how many of us engage in this kind of "speed sleeping," it is questionable whether insufficient sleep syndrome is truly voluntary or a basic requirement of modern life. In spite of devastating effects on health, productivity, and welfare, speed sleeping appears to have become the norm.

Consequently, millions of us routinely struggle with sleepiness and fatigue throughout the day. Our chronic sleep debt has spawned an industry, if not an entire lifestyle, devoted to enhancing personal energy through stimulating substances and activities that effectively mask our debilitating sleepiness. Coffee and black teas are the most commonly consumed beverages on earth. And antidepressant medications, particularly SSRIs and related drugs, believed by some experts to be not much more than medically sanctioned stimulants, are now prescribed in record numbers to keep us from sagging throughout the day.

Bill missed his work as a long-haul trucker since his license was revoked following a second vehicular mishap attributed to his falling asleep at the wheel. Bill's head was heavy, distracting him again from his resolve to take a bite out of the stacks of overdue paperwork all around him. Despite getting more than ten hours of sleep the night before, he still struggled to stay alert and focused on his task. He took a bite out of the pastry stashed in his top left drawer instead. But it reminded him of the bargain he had made with his wife. Once he got caught up on work, he would try to diet and exercise again. She was rightly concerned, given that his physician thought his high blood pressure was weight related. Bill's heart was heavy, too. He wondered when his new antidepressant medication would finally kick in.

Unfortunately, Bill is not alone. According to the National Sleep Foundation (2005), 60 percent of American adult drivers acknowledge that they have driven a motor vehicle when feeling drowsy within the past year. Four percent had an accident or near accident in the past year because of sleepiness or dozing off while driving. Among this group, 29 percent report having had an accident or near accident at least monthly over the past year. About one-third of this group (37 percent) report that they have nodded off or fallen asleep while driving a vehicle, even just for a brief moment. Among these respondents, 13 percent say they have done so at least once a month. Conservative estimates by the National Highway Traffic Safety Administration (2005) suggest that 100,000 police-reported automobile crashes are the direct result of driver fatigue each year. These crashes result in an estimated 1,550 deaths and 71,000 injuries. But these estimates are believed to be the tip of the iceberg, since it is difficult to ascertain if sleep deprivation was the cause of an automobile accident.

Chronic daytime sleepiness is known to significantly compromise productivity and competence across all trades and professions. According to the National Commission on Sleep Disorders Research (1998), the annual cost of sleep-related problems in the United States is estimated to be $50 to $100 billion. And then there are the medical and emotional costs to the millions of people who, like Bill, suffer from undiagnosed obstructive sleep apnea. Given Bill's deeply deluded belief that he sleeps quite well, his doctors attributed his growing fatigue to depression and being overweight. And Bill continues to plod through his days dazed and dangerous.

Larry sat fidgeting in his therapist's waiting room, anxious about being late again. He had been up most of the night studying for an anthropology midterm with the help of four mugs of black coffee. Later, he tried to get some sleep by drinking a few beers. At twenty-seven, Larry had struggled with attention deficit disorder (ADD) for most of his life. A chronic sense of failure and low self-esteem brought him back to therapy.

Dr. Crone stepped into the waiting room, looking puzzled.

"Oh, hi . . . Hi, Dr. Crone," Larry exclaimed. "I'm really sorry . . . about being late. I mean . . . you see, I—"

Dr. Crone interrupted. "Larry, it's Tuesday. I have you down for our regular Thursday appointment." Larry's face flushed with shame, a shame laced with self-loathing and hopelessness. Here was further confirmation that he would never escape the chronic chaos that engulfed his life.

As a young adult Larry continued fighting an underlying depression with various prescription medications and illicit drugs. But his life continued to spin out of control and back into chaos and confusion. He seemed to cycle from energy born of dramatic emotional reactions to the burnout of fatigue.

After a number of sessions, Dr. Crone remained perplexed about assigning a primary diagnosis to Larry. Beyond his ADD, there were clearly signs of an anxiety disorder. Could he be bipolar? Larry also reported chronic insufficient and fitful sleep. Sometimes this was due to drug use, but more often the drug use seemed to be a sad, boggled attempt at self-medicating his restlessness and insomnia. Larry's life seemed a magnet for crisis and drama. Dr. Crone had seen a number of other patients like this and wondered about creating a new diagnostic category for adrenaline addiction.

Sleep and Dream Deprivation

Although Mary, Bill, and Larry come from diverse backgrounds and struggle with markedly different sleep disorders, they share lives mired in chronic sleep and dream debt, sustained by counterfeit energies, and shrouded in deep denial. Unaware of the extent of their damaged night consciousness and the ensuing daytime daze, they routinely struggle with disorientation, depression, and even dangerousness. Their lives remain embedded in the ubiquitous daze that envelops our world.

Sleep and dream debt is cumulative. Most of us have experienced the occasional loss of part or all of a night's sleep; we are aware of the physical and emotional toll it takes. What few people realize is that unpaid sleep and dream debt accumulates over time, profoundly affecting our waking consciousness.

Sleep and dream deprivation is *disorienting*. Research confirms that it distorts our perception, impairs our judgment, and disrupts our behavior. When we are drowsy, we are also apt to experience recurring *microsleeps*. These are sudden, unconscious flashes of sleep, lasting for a few seconds to a minute, which can occur with our eyes wide open. Sleepiness and fatigue are associated with blunted senses, a general slowing of mental processes, memory deficits, and otherwise compromised cognitive abilities. Being disoriented renders us dysfunctional in many subtle and not so subtle ways. Some experts even believe that the distractedness symptomatic of attention deficit disorder may be associated with chronic sleep deprivation.

Given that the very essence of depression is diminished energy, how could chronic sleep and dream deprivation not be a critical factor in the epidemic of clinical depression that plagues our world today? Although insomnia is known to be a common symptom of depression, we saw earlier that depression was also a very common outcome of chronic insomnia. One year of insomnia significantly increases one's chance of becoming clinically depressed. The incidence of depression is also significantly increased among people with obstructive sleep apnea. Given what we know about the strong connection between chronic sleep and dream deprivation and mood disturbances, many of us might just be better off napping on our psychotherapist's couch.

Disorientation and depression are associated with significant decrements in work performance and staggering increases in all sorts of accidents. "Eventually, if the sleep debt becomes large enough," warns sleep psychologist Stanley Coren, "we become clumsy, stupid, unhappy, and dead" (1996, 11). From truck drivers to airline pilots and students to surgeons, no one is immune to the detrimental effects of sleep deprivation.

The cartoon icon Homer Simpson, often depicted asleep at his job at the Springfield nuclear power plant, is frighteningly close to reality. As a group, nuclear power plant night shift workers suffer from excessive sleepiness and fatigue. More than half of all shift workers fall asleep on the job at least once a week (National Commission on Sleep Disorders Research, 2005). There is evidence that the Three Mile Island, Chernobyl, Bhopal, and *Exxon Valdez* disasters were all related to sleep deprivation.

Traffic hazards due to sleepiness are comparable to those resulting from drunken driving. Research in this area suggests that there is little difference between driving drowsy and driving drunk. It is a mistake, however, to limit this comparison only to driving. There simply is not much difference between being chronically sleep deprived and being intoxicated. Fortunately, we are beginning to see the enactment of laws to protect the public against drowsy driving.

I believe that the denial of our pernicious and ubiquitous sleep and dream deprivation may be the greatest consensual pretense of our times. Since sleep and dream deprivation compromises our perceptual abilities, our ability to clearly perceive the impact of our own sleepiness is also diminished. Disturbed perception will readily mask itself. When we do not see clearly, we do not see clearly that we do not see clearly.

Compensating with Counterfeit Energies

Our debilitating daze is further complicated by a semiconscious pattern of dependence on counterfeit energies that mask our depletion. We routinely seek out excessive daytime stimulation to counter our excessive daytime sleepiness. Too often we confuse the need for rest or sleep with a need for coffee, a cigarette, or pound cake—or a quick infusion of drama-mediated adrenaline. These are counterfeit energies simply because they are not what they appear to be. They spike up sharply, giving us a false, temporary sense of power that, unlike more natural energies, cannot be sustained. And then they quickly backfire, leaving us even more depleted, jittery, and in need of another fix.

When we need to function despite our chronic sleep and dream debt, we reflexively seek out sources of quick energy for symptomatic relief. In addition to the common overindulgence in caffeine and refined sugars, I believe we also unknowingly depend heavily on adrenaline. And as we have previously discussed, our dependence on excessive LAN serves as a ready nightly backup.

Sugar

Sugar is the basic source of fuel for our bodies and brains. Most natural forms of sugar break down gradually in the body, releasing a fairly even flow of energy. Like throwing a piece of hardwood on the fire, natural sugars burn more steadily. Our diets today, however, are rich in refined sugars, which are absorbed rapidly, resulting in a burst of energy. This is more like throwing newspaper on the fire. Our energies flare up but then die down just as rapidly.

As a society, we are dependent on processed carbohydrates— white breads, white rice, and white sugars. And we love our refined sugary snacks, our cakes, candy bars, and ice cream. "Sugar consumption is off the charts," states Michael F. Jacobson, executive director of the Center for Science in the Public Interest (CSPI). He points out that sugary foods now account for about 15 to 20 percent of our caloric intake, a rise of about 10 percent over the past twenty-five years. According to the CSPI, soft drinks are consistently the best-selling product in American grocery stores. The U.S. Department of Agriculture estimates that, on average, Americans consume about twice as much sugar every day as is recommended (CSPI 1998). We burn empty calories throughout the day with the same abandon that we burn gasoline in our cars.

Soft drinks, affectionately known as "liquid candy," are a major source of increased sugar consumption around the world. The average twelve-ounce can of soda contains about ten teaspoons, or forty grams, of refined sugars. Per capita consumption of soft drinks in the United States has increased about sevenfold in the past sixty years. In fact, the average American now consumes more than fifty gallons of soft drinks each year, primarily the caffeinated variety (CSPI 2005). And as generations of pop commercials promise, these fluids will antidote our daze by restoring youth and excitement to our lives.

Although most soft drinks have considerably less caffeine than coffee (there are some striking exceptions), research has shown that a single can of soda contains sufficient caffeine to produce measurable mood and behavioral changes, including irritability, anxiety, and restlessness. These changes have been compared to classic symptoms of anxiety neuroses, a condition that is, in part, characterized by excessive energy.

When our energy dips, particularly if it does so suddenly, we reflexively seek to replenish it. Scientific evidence indicates that the need to rest or sleep can easily become confused with the need to eat. Interestingly, the biochemical messengers that inform the brain and body of the need to sleep are the same ones that communicate hunger. Given pressures to be productive, on the one hand, and the ready availability of energy-spiking sugary foods and drinks, on the other, many people confuse being tired or sleepy with being hungry. By raising blood sugar levels, eating can at least temporarily mask our need to rest or sleep.

Caffeine

In a historic act of rebellion against escalating British taxes on tea, a group of disguised colonists dumped a large shipment of the stuff into the Boston harbor in 1774. Tea was out. And almost overnight drinking coffee became a symbol of American patriotism and freedom. Cup for cup, coffee has three times more caffeine than tea does. We showed the British.

The founding fathers proceeded to draft their strategies to liberate a new nation—in coffeehouses. Members of the Continental Congress first read the Declaration of Independence aloud to the public at Merchant's Coffee House in Philadelphia. Little did they know that they were also establishing a tradition that would shape our lifestyles and identities in a profound way for centuries to come. Caffeine, particularly in the form of coffee, has become an integral part of our culture and our selves. As David Letterman once put it, "If it wasn't for coffee, I would have no discernible personality at all" (Zehme 1994). Millions of people laughed. Nervously.

Caffeine, found in coffee, tea, many soft drinks, chocolate products, and a variety of medications, is our world's most popular drug. The National Coffee Association (2000) reports that 54 percent of the U.S. adult population drinks coffee daily, while an additional 25 percent of Americans drink coffee occasionally. We consume approximately four hundred cups of coffee—or over twenty-six gallons—per capita each year (National Coffee Association 2000). Between 80 and 90 percent of us consume caffeine in one form or another every single day. And we are not alone. As an international commodity, coffee is second only to oil. And these statistics do not account for the caffeine we get from teas, soft drinks, and other caffeinated beverages.

Caffeine, particularly in the form of coffee, is the primary fuel for the vehicle of our personal drive. It is our traditional "leaded" gasoline. More popular than nicotine and alcohol, caffeine is deeply integrated into the fabric of modern life and readily accessible. Witness the explosive growth of Starbucks shops around the world, not to mention their innumerous clones.

Despite the fact that it is a fairly potent drug with complex properties and widespread influences on our biological and psychological functioning, caffeine still remains completely unregulated. Given the broad and uncertain range of its medical implications, if caffeine were introduced as a new drug today, experts agree that it simply would not meet with FDA approval.

The period of active influence of a drug or chemical in the body is measured in terms of its half-life, the amount of time it takes the body to metabolize about one-half of the substance in our blood. The half-life of caffeine can vary from several hours to several days. For a nonsmoking adult the effects can last from about five to seven hours. Various medications, the use of oral contraceptives, and pregnancy can significantly lengthen the half-life of caffeine. Grapefruit contains a substance called naringin, which also increases the half-life of caffeine. Cigarette smoking reduces the half-life of caffeine to about three hours, probably contributing to smokers consuming more coffee than nonsmokers.

Though many people argue that they drink coffee because they "love the taste," it is more likely that caffeine is popular because it serves as a potent stimulant. It speeds up metabolism, raises blood pressure and heart rate, and accelerates breathing. It also can temporarily offset the effects of sleep and dream deprivation. Although sensitivity to caffeine varies widely, doses ranging from 250 to 750 mg (about two to seven cups of coffee) can result in restlessness, disturbed sleep, tension, and even cardiac arrhythmias.

Caffeine increases the release of adrenaline, which increases alertness and in sufficient quantities can cause varying degrees of a fight-or-flight reaction. Contrary to popular opinion, caffeine does not literally provide us with extra energy; it primarily masks our experience of depletion—of our need to rest. Adenosine is a natural by-product of the body's burning of fuel, a kind of recyclable exhaust. As available energy supplies are used up, adenosine levels rise, reach a threshold, and trigger special receptors in the brain that signal the experience of sleepiness. When caffeine is ingested, it quickly binds with these same receptors, blocking their sensitivity to adenosine. Consequently, the message of exhaustion then does not reach the brain and body. We are sleepy but do not get the signal. Caffeine does not provide us with more fuel—it essentially damages our fuel gauge, misleading us into thinking we are not running on empty.

Recent studies have determined that caffeine also suppresses melatonin. Given the critical role of melatonin in maintaining general health and promoting sleep and dreams, I believe we need to seriously reconsider the nonchalant attitude with which we regularly consume this potent drug.

Gratuitous Drama

Our culture's obvious attraction to gratuitous drama—all things exciting and hyperbolic—also functions to generate energy by increasing the release of adrenaline. *Exciting* has become a synonym for all things good. Whether we are talking about people, films, or foods, if it is worth experiencing, it is exciting. We are a culture with an insatiable appetite for excitement, particularly in the form of the dramatic.

We probably all know people who qualify as drama queens. But a more subtle and pervasive kind of drama now permeates ordinary daily life, reflected in peculiar hyperbole, hair triggers, misplaced angst, and epidemic hypertension that we accept as the norm. Witness most of what passes for the "news"—hyperbolic sound bites of gratuitous calamity, disaster, disease, war, and political intrigue. In my professional work, I am frequently struck by the prevalent use of terms like *urgency* and *emergency* in our daily lives.

Drama is gratuitous excitement. Dramatic thoughts, feelings, and behaviors trigger the release of adrenaline, which provides an instantaneous rush of energy that will temporarily counter our depletion. I believe that many people confuse this rush of emotional energy with genuine meaning and value.

Drama distracts us through a kind of neurotic excessiveness, a psychological sleight of hand that calls our attention away from what is truly meaningful. Carl Jung taught that *all neurosis is an excuse for legitimate suffering*. Drama serves to temporarily protect us from the legitimate suffering associated with being depleted and dazed.

Chronic sleep and dream deprivation predisposes us to perceive, think, and act in ways that stimulate the compensatory overproduction of adrenaline. Gratuitous drama offers a temporary, quick fix for daze, but like sugar and caffeine, it eventually backfires.

LAN as Counterfeit Energy

Beyond sugar, caffeine, and adrenaline, perhaps the most insidious form of our energy dependence is on excessive light at night (LAN). As we have seen, exposure to even relatively low levels of light at night can energize us sufficiently to delay our sleep phase and bedtime. Not only has LAN freed us from the constraints of natural circadian rhythms, it has also become a major source of counterfeit energy.

Effectively, we are all under social pressure to be "night people." So much of the good life in modern times is available only by night. Whether we declare ourselves night owls or not, if we choose to partake of life in any normal fashion, we are expected to be up well into darkness on a regular basis. I believe that in nature, however, there are no true night people. From a biological perspective, we evolved to be awake and active by day and resting and asleep by night. Whether we consider ourselves night owls or larks, I believe that, by nature, we are all morning people.

So-called night people are those who have learned to seek out extra energies at night. In my work with many self-proclaimed night owls, I have consistently observed their strong and often unconscious tendency to utilize counterfeit energies in the evening— a bowl of chocolate ice cream, a murder mystery, an exciting work project, a last-chance fight with their partner, a cup of coffee, and, of course, a very well-lit room. Despite protests on the part of night owls that they are naturally aroused at night, virtually all of them are drawn to various sources of light at night.

Artificial Waking

Coffee drinks are getting stronger, sugar consumption continues to skyrocket, the use of stimulating antidepressants is increasing dramatically, and adrenaline-mediated drama is at play everywhere. But we are still wilting. Perhaps we are habituating to these forms of counterfeit energies and now need even harder stuff.

Among sleep medicine's most disturbing recent developments is a misplaced excitement about the promise of artificial waking. Newer types of stimulant drugs that have less of the uncomfortable speedy side effects of older stimulants are being touted as the great hope for managing excessive sleepiness. The real excitement about such medicines, however, is more about their potential to help us overcome our very need for rest and sleep.

Modafinil, also known as Provigil, is one such drug that has obtained FDA approval for treating the excessive daytime sleepiness associated with narcolepsy and hypersomnia. Almost from the start, however, this medication was being extensively prescribed for off-label use, that is, for treating various other causes of sleepiness and fatigue. Increasing numbers of prescriptions for Modafinil are being written to "treat" the daytime symptoms of insomnia and apnea, as well as to treat fatigue due to other causes. Not surprisingly, the drug has become a popular treatment for attention deficit disorders as well. Perhaps most disturbing are reports of growing numbers of people who do not have sleep disorders but are using Modafinil to help them function with less sleep.

Although SSRI antidepressants are not commonly thought of as stimulants, they do have a stimulating effect upon the brain. Producing substantial increases in neurotransmitters like serotonin, they increase our subjective sense of energy. But given the extended half-life of most of these drugs, their stimulating effect remains active throughout the night, potentially damaging our sleep. The use of Prozac, for example, is associated with increases in sleep onset latency, decreased deep sleep, and compromised dreaming.

Just as we have grown accustomed to thinking about taking something for sleep, we are beginning to think more and more about taking something for waking. Waking pills, whether in the form of stimulating antidepressants or the new generation of stimulant medications, essentially mask our daytime daze and further damage the quality of our sleep and dreams at night. Like sleeping pills, which do not result in true, natural sleep, I believe waking pills mask our damaged daytime consciousness with artificial, relentless alertness. The half-life of waking pills varies from twelve to fifteen hours for Modafinil to as much as seven days for stimulating antidepressants like Prozac. Whether we are aware of it or not, these medications are likely maintaining a substantial energy buzz in our brains around the clock. Such background noise inevitably erodes the quality of our sleep and dreams, not to mention our circadian rhythms.

Dampened Daylight

In addition to being obviously sleep and dream deprived, we are also chronically wake deprived. After failing to fully surrender to the dark of night, many of us never fully awaken to the light of day. And just as our failure to descend deeply into night adversely affects our days, our limited ascension into day also damages our nights.

It is one of the great ironies of modern life that we frantically grope for counterfeit energies while shunning our primary source of natural energy—the sun. Natural sunlight energizes and orients us in remarkable ways that science is just beginning to understand. Earlier we saw that sunlight suspends the production of melatonin, resets the body clock, and stimulates the release of serotonin.

Just as we shun natural darkness, we routinely shield ourselves from sunlight. It is as if some of the darkness we have stolen from night sneaks back to reclaim some of our day. We stay indoors, in the shade, behind our curtains, blinds, and tinted windows. We typically work, play, and otherwise live indoors. We are a culture of solar phobics, content to live out the bulk of our lives indoors, proud to sport our protective sunglasses, sun block, and other sun gear, even during periods of little or no solar risk. Despite the fact that the sun has been revered as a source of sacred and healing energies for thousands of years, physicians today are more concerned with its dangers than its possibilities.

Because morning sun is the most potent of zeitgebers, our solar dampening most likely damages our circadian rhythms. As we saw previously, light stimulates the release of serotonin and can be used as an effective treatment for different kinds of depression. Conversely, we know that extended exposure to low light conditions is a factor in seasonal affective disorders. Since natural sunlight both energizes and orients us, shielding ourselves from it further contributes to the blunting of our waking consciousness.

"People were designed to be outside," writes sleep specialist Daniel Kripke. "Our modern human ancestors became intelligent in places which were indeed very sunny. It is for such a life that our bodies are adapted" (2002). Throughout most of human history, most of life was lived outdoors. Even when humans migrated to less hospitable climates, they still spent significantly more time outside than we do. Over recent decades "civilized" people have migrated indoors and are spending significantly less time in natural outdoor light. Indoor environments continue to grow more comfortable, functional, and entertaining, further discouraging our spending time outdoors.

Kripke and his colleagues determined that adults living in San Diego spent an average of less than one hour per day outdoors. Although some people spent significantly more time outside each day, many others actually spent only ten to twenty minutes in natural light (Kripke 2002). Given that San Diego has a hospitable year-round climate, people in other locales may be spending even less time outdoors.

The intensity of light or illumination is commonly measured in terms of "lux." A candle that is one foot away from an object will cast one *foot-candle* of light onto that object. This is the equivalent of about 10 lux.

Direct sunlight can reach and even exceed 100,000 lux, while indirect sunlight on a clear day can provide up to 20,000 lux. Within a few minutes after sunrise on a clear spring or fall morning, illumination reaches 10,000 lux. In contrast, an overcast day may provide only 1,000 lux. An exceptionally well-lit office provides about 500 lux, while a conventionally lit room at home provides about 300 to 400 lux.

Outside, twilight provides about 10 lux, a full moon measures at 0.1 lux, a moonless clear night sky a mere 0.001 lux, and a moonless overcast night sky a dark 0.0001 lux. Generally speaking, it is significantly brighter outside than it is indoors during daylight hours. At night, however, it is significantly brighter indoors than it is outside.

Instead of availing ourselves of natural light by day, we head indoors and become overexposed to dampened artificial light. Natural light is gently rhythmic. The sun metes out a broad dynamic tempo as it traverses the sky. Artificial light does not; it is monotonous and relentless—apropos for our driven lifestyles.

For too many people today, a common source of daytime rhythmicity is the stroboscopic flicker of fluorescent lights over their workstations. I believe we routinely overdose on fluorescents, incandescents, halogens, and neon. According to John Ott, who spent decades researching the relationship of health and light, this kind of artificial light takes its toll, compromising our health, well-being, and productivity.

Our conundrum with light is strikingly parallel to our dilemma with food. As a nation, we are overfed, yet undernourished. We consume too many calories, but since so many of them are "empty," we remain nutrient deficient. Likewise, with regard to light, we consume too much artificial, "junk" light but remain deficient in our exposure to natural and naturally timed light.

BRAC: The Rest of Our Daily Lives

Bob Dylan once said, "There are no rest stops on the highway of life." This certainly holds true for life in our modern world, where genuine rest is so devalued. In my travels, I have noticed many highway rest stops where the only place to sit and rest outside of one's automobile was the restroom. Restrooms are aptly named since they are probably the most common place of rest during the workday. At one highway rest stop in southern Arizona, I discovered a large sign that actually provided a list of instructions for how to use the area. The very first instruction read, "Rest and relax." Yes, we do need to be told.

As an alternative to life in a daze, a more lucid approach to waking calls for a deeper understanding of BRAC, the basic rest and activity cycles introduced in chapter 2. If we let them, these natural speed bumps of waking life can help us reinstate a missing sense of rhythm into our waking day, balancing our incessant drive with encouragement to slow down and rest.

BRAC is the common rhythmic matrix of the process of sleep and waking. We saw earlier that our sleep cycles are structured by ninety-minute ultradian rhythms. As these same ultradian rhythms continue to cycle into and through the day, they are referred to as BRAC. BRAC provides the basic structure for most psychological and biological processes, ranging from cellular activity to cyclic changes in consciousness. Like the rhythmic roll of ocean waves, our energies gradually swell and rise, reach their crest, and then recede. As its name implies, BRAC specifically regulates the fundamental balance of activity and rest. BRAC is about the rhythmic beckoning of *rest* throughout our waking day.

Beyond the compelling call of the restroom, many of us simply do not attend to more subtle signals to cease activity. BRAC is nature's rest stop, advising us of when and even how to rest. The major portion of each ninety-minute BRAC period is characterized by what we might consider ordinary waking consciousness. It supports our being attentive, focused, and productive. We are then invited into a respite in subtle but unmistakable ways. We get distracted, find ourselves looking out the window, daydreaming, yawning, and stretching. Our attention shifts inward to the body, where we might notice some thirst, hunger, a change in body temperature, or a call to the restroom. The remaining twenty minutes of each BRAC period, then, breaks us away from ordinary activity, entailing a shift to a more relaxed and expansive consciousness. As we will see in chapter 9, BRAC invites us into the waking dream. Ernest Rossi refers to the resting portion of the BRAC process as the *ultradian healing response.*

Rest is indeed healing because it allows us a few moments to recoup our energy, relax our focus, and reorient to our interior. During this ultradian dip, our energy output is slowed; we cool down and turn inward. Our focus becomes relaxed, and we drop into a diffuse, waking, dreamlike consciousness—a kind of reverie. As we rest, the basic frame of our perception loosens, and a broader vista appears. We become the artist dropping back to evaluate our painting. We reorient, lifting above the trees of our close-up, ordinary perception to glimpse again the forest of possibilities all around us.

Most of us have no difficulty with the active, energized aspect of the BRAC wave. But because of our myopic industrious focus, we miss and resist the ultradian healing response. We have seen that our overly industrious expectations reinforce the use of counterfeit energies to keep us going. We bound mindlessly over our energy dips in an effort to operate like machines, like cars over speed bumps, like our heroic Energizer Bunny.

We would rather not slow down because rest allows suppressed negative emotions to surface. In chapter 2, I discussed the common confusion of rest with various activities, getting high, and entertainment. These ways of redefining rest simply render it inert. When we slow down, we are likely to come back to our bodies and ourselves. We are more prone to feel, to experience our emotions—another dreaded possibility for the opportunistic emergence of shadowy material—by day no less.

Many people feel anxious as they start to slow down, and they jump to the conclusion that this anxiety results from their slowing. They believe they become anxious because there is much that still needs to be done. Others have a vague sense that slowing down and resting are somehow wrong. We have all learned that the devil makes work for idle hands. In actuality, this anxiety is a sign of opportunistic emergence. And we typically kill the messenger. When we do not allow ourselves to rest, to dip, to fully plunge, we fail to rebound, to resurge, to be fully awake. The naturally robust cycles of activity and rest, like a microcosm of our wake and sleep cycles, become flattened.

The ultradian healing response is not about the classic coffee break in a small florescent room with metal furniture and vending machines. It may well include a visit to the restroom and maybe even to the kitchen for a sensible snack. It might also be about sitting down, lying down, letting go, stretching, meditating, or giving free rein to one's imagination. The ultradian healing response is about consciously and intentionally allowing ourselves to rest when we feel the need.

BRAC encourages us to bring more awareness to the rhythmic structure of our waking lives. In consistently bounding over our BRAC, we lose control of the day. Taking regular rest breaks helps us modulate the speed of our runaway lives and prevents us from a head-on collision with night. The secret of a good night's sleep is, indeed, a good day's waking. And other than attending to BRAC, one of the most effective ways I know of modulating our waking pace, of creating a really good day's waking, is through the regular practice of napping.

A Note on Napping

> You must sleep sometime between lunch and dinner, and no halfway measures. Take off your clothes and get into bed. That's what I always do. Don't think you will be doing less work because you sleep during the day. That's a foolish notion held by people who

have no imaginations. You will be able to accomplish
more. You get two days in one—well, at least one and
a half. (As quoted in Maas 1998)

This famous comment by Winston Churchill made over a half-
century ago summarizes what science has since been confirming
about napping. We are biologically programmed to nap. In addition to our regular BRAC dips in energy, we experience a drop in
body temperature in the afternoon that is designed to encourage
us to sleep, independently of our nighttime sleeping patterns.

Churchill's neighbors in the Mediterranean, as well as people
in Latin American cultures, have long indulged in a sweet tradition of afternoon naps. Americans, on the other hand, have had an
almost pathological view of regular napping. Although few people
would likely argue against daily napping in principle, most do in
practice. The average American adult takes only one to two naps
per week, while 25 percent never nap at all (Maas 1998). Unless
you are a young child or elderly, daytime sleeping will likely be
viewed as a sign of illness, laziness, or substance use.

Unfortunately, we are more apt to respond to our midafternoon
slump by trying to jump-start ourselves with counterfeit energies.
Such strategies only mask our underlying depletion, further depriving us of the rest and sleep we need. As an alternative, a brief afternoon nap will restore our natural energy, help reactivate our brains,
and improve our ability to focus. Progressive companies that offer
their employees an opportunity to nap during the workday have
found that it reduces accidents, improves productivity, and enhances
morale. Sleep scientists believe that naps taken in the middle of our
waking day provide greater benefit than adding that same amount of
sleep time to our nightly slumber. "Napping should not be frowned
upon at the office or make you feel guilty at home," states James
Maas. "It should have the status of daily exercise" (1998, 108).

Napping is a social statement. It asserts that rest and sleep are
important, equally important to wakefulness and productivity. One's
willingness and ability to sleep by day is also a reflection of one's
valuation of sleep by night. Napping is also a psychological state-

ment. It is essential to balancing the day's powerful call to extraversion with a remembrance of our inner self. Naps can lighten our spirits, as well. Yogi Berra, a devout napper, said "I usually take a two-hour nap from 1:00 p.m. until 4:00 p.m." Naps take us out of time, out of day time, providing a dash of night consciousness in the midst of our waking day. Just as "night watch" may reflect the light center in the dark, night wave of the yin-yang, napping may be the dark center of the white, waking wave of the yin-yang.

Lucid Waking Practices

Simply having our eyes open does not necessarily mean we are fully awake. Consider using the following practices to help you become more fully aware throughout the day.

Determine Your Daze

Try to become more cognizant of any personal daze you might have and the habits that might be reinforcing it. Evaluate your use of counterfeit energies, and plan to gradually diminish these over a reasonable period of time. Consider how daze might be functional in your life. Think about how you might experience your life with a clearer mind and naturally energized body.

Practice tuning into your personal energy levels by installing a virtual gauge that you regularly check. Notice the natural fluctuations in your energy. How do you react when you begin to feel a bit weary? Notice what you tell yourself about dips in your energy. And notice how you deal with them. Let yourself be mindful of your thoughts and feelings when you feel fatigued or sleepy during the day. Notice any judgments you may have about this.

Be Mindful of Counterfeit Energizers

Consider charting your use of counterfeit energies for a week or two. Make note of your caffeine consumption, use of refined sugars, and attraction to dramatic experiences. Try to become more aware of the kinds of thoughts, feelings, sensations, and experiences that serve as a cue for your seeking such energies. Also, notice your reactions to the use of such energies, especially how they leave you feeling as they wear off.

Take BRAC Breaks

Tune into and practice regular BRAC breaks through the day. Be mindful of the common signals of the start of your ultradian healing response. Notice when you become distracted, begin to stretch and yawn, or become dreamy. Also notice when your attention is drawn inward to any bodily needs.

Temporarily let go of the activity you are engaged in and experiment with simple ways of restfully meeting your needs at these times. Consider a moment of meditation, some deep breathing, a gentle walk, or some stretching. Let your focus broaden, allowing your thinking to become more loose, abstract, and artistic. Also become mindful of any feelings, needs, and wants lingering in the background. You might visualize yourself panning back from the momentary picture of your life to obtain a larger vista. Let yourself indulge in whatever restful experiences call to you for about twenty minutes or until you feel a natural return of your energy.

Pay Off Your Sleep and Dream Debt

The simplest way to pay off a sleep debt is to give yourself an extended period of time during which you sleep for as long as you wish every night. Consider taking at least a week, and perhaps up to three or more weeks, in which you arrange your daily schedule to allow for this. Obviously, for most people, this is more easily accomplished on vacation.

During this period, follow the recommendations offered in previous chapters for promoting healthy sleep, particularly those about dusk simulation. You will probably notice an increase in your total nightly sleep time as your body compensates for previously lost sleep and dreams. Try to maintain an open-ended sleep schedule until your sleep debt is fully paid off.

Consider Napping

Experiment with introducing regular midday naps into your life. For most people, this presents a challenge to ordinary work or household schedules. Keep in mind that napping offers distinct benefits to our personal and work lives.

I like Winston Churchill's advice about getting out of one's day clothes and into bed when possible. If this is impractical, a couch, a recliner, or any other comfortable spot will do. Take brief naps of twenty to thirty minutes as close to the middle of your waking day as you can. (Long and late-afternoon naps take us into deeper sleep, can result in extended grogginess, and can shift our circadian rhythms, compromising the quality of our nighttime sleep.) Make napping a daily practice, allowing yourself to rest with your eyes closed even if you do not feel like sleeping.

Tempting as they may be, naps are generally contraindicated for people who have insomnia, since they can further diminish nighttime sleep. On the other hand, napping is especially helpful for people trying to heal from illness or injury.

～

Waking is the internal representation of daylight. Unfortunately, many of us are wake deprived and unaware of it. We live in a chronic daze clouded by sleep and dream debt, dependence on counterfeit energies, and excessive shielding from natural daylight. In the end, we find that elements of night are essential to heal our days. Just as there are subtle aspects of light permeating night and darkness, there are subtle aspects of night and darkness woven into the background of the day as BRAC rest periods and our inclination to nap.

⌒ 8

Shadow: Making Peace with Night

One does not become enlightened by imagining figures of light, but by making the darkness conscious. The latter procedure, however, is disagreeable and therefore not popular.

—CARL G. JUNG

"NOW, BREATHE IN DEEPLY . . . inhale this clarity, the grace and healing that's all around us. Hold the breath for just a moment as you completely absorb these blessings ... and, once again, release ... exhaling all the darkness, fear, and pain within ... just letting it go."

I sat as cross-legged as I could on the floor of a small, simple meditation room with about twenty other participants in this weekend spiritual retreat at a beautiful ranch just outside of Los Angeles. Our instructor, Angela, an attractive and accomplished psychotherapist and yoga teacher, was gently guiding us through a series of visualizations and breathing exercises designed to quiet the mind, soothe the body, and promote psychological healing. It was the early eighties, the heyday of the spiritual *sweetness and light* movement.

"And once more now," she continued, "very slowly let yourself inhale deeply ... gratefully receiving all of the wondrous, healing energy you deserve ... And now ... squeezing as much air as you can out of your lungs, exhale all the remaining darkness, anxiety, and pain from within . . . just breathe them out . . . releasing them completely."

Although I had participated in similar programs before and derived benefit from them, I noticed a vague sense of uneasiness on this particular day. When we repeated the same exercise the next morning, my attention expanded beyond my personal experience to envision the other people around me. I saw them inhaling goodness, light, and healing, then exhaling darkness, pain, and anxiety—all into the room we were sharing. I sensed the room filling with murky psychic refuse, becoming polluted with spiritual smog. I found myself growing reluctant to breathe at all, let alone take another deep breath.

We toss our litter into the street, whether blatantly around our neighborhoods and natural environments or, cleverly veiled in spiritual or religious pursuit, through the thoughtless projection of our personal darkness into the invisible world. We witness everywhere a pattern of consuming all that seems sweet and good and discarding the containers the stuff came in. We deny, repress, suppress, and project our fears and anxieties—our darkness and our shadows—as a routine part of everyday life. They are projected out the doors of our perception, tossed into our neighbors' yards, or smuggled across spiritual state lines. Like radioactive waste, some of the most dangerous things we discard slowly fester in the background, hurting our communities, our families, our children, our planet, and ourselves.

Our disturbed relationship with night is ultimately rooted in our discomfort with and denial of the dark side of our own selves. To heal night, we must heal our relationship to darkness, both as an environmental state and as its internal analogue—the psychospiritual experience of *shadow*. But we demonstrate great personal and public reluctance to acknowledge and address shadow issues, to take responsibility for and clean up our own psychological refuse. This reluctance and denial inevitably sneak back to haunt us in the form of night's many nemeses.

The word *night* was derived originally from the goddess Nyx, who was the sister of Erebus, the embodiment of primordial darkness, and also the mother of Doom, Nemesis, Retribution, and Strife. Understandably, *night* has a secondary meaning. It refers to *a condition or time of obscurity, sinfulness, or misfortune*. Night is a natural medium for shadow. We have a primordial fear of night and its darkness, which seems simultaneously to inhibit and disinhibit us.

Darkness is a naturally inhibitory force in the lives of diurnal beings. We discussed the slowing influence of dusk and the quieting effect of night in earlier chapters. Since we lose the visual information we depend so heavily on to define our behaviors and ourselves, we get lost in the dark. Obviously, in more primitive settings we would face the risk of unseen dangers lurking in the night. But even in modern times night is known to host more than its share of accidents, injuries, and attacks.

The night is rife with nemeses. It harbors an assortment of "bad" people—from ordinary drunks, burglars, and prostitutes to terrorists, murderers, and the insane. Most nocturnal animals, such as owls, bats, and rats, have developed dubious reputations given their association with dire forebodings, blood thirst, and contagion. Worse yet are werewolves, ghosts, bogeymen, vampires, and other supernatural beings that haunt the night.

But night and darkness also free us from our daytime constraints. We become disinhibited by night. It is as if night is a spiritual duty-free zone. There are things we do under the cover of darkness that we suspect even angels cannot see. If the day is the province of public, the night is highly personal. Nighttime has its own conventions that offer us greater personal license. While the social expectations of day tell us how we should be, night reveals all of who we really are. We take off our clothes at night. In loosening social constraints, night allows our shadows to emerge. Darkness inhibits us because it disinhibits us.

The Repression of Shadow

I have stressed the critical role of the opportunistic emergence of anxieties and shadow issues in understanding night consciousness, including sleeping and dreaming. Night becomes a repository for denied and repressed waking issues. Resistance of daytime rest and nighttime slowing obscures awareness of our interiors, emotions, anxieties, and, particularly, our shadow.

Avoidance of BRAC breaks and naps prevents our shadows from breathing throughout the day. We then buffer our encounter with dusk and darkness by failing to slow and naturally surrender to night. Excessive nighttime illumination both energizes us and literally lights the way for maintaining an active daytime frame of mind into the night. Whatever else artificial evening light does, it damages social structures that support us in regularly processing our shadow issues. Our collective avoidance of shadow issues is associated with a peculiar social trend sometimes referred to as "light chasing."

Light chasing refers to our contemporary inclination to deny the existence of darkness and the need for addressing shadow. It is associated with a Pollyannaish, runaway "positive thinking" approach evident in much pop psychology and spirituality today. This light-chasing philosophy was recently brought to public attention by Debbie Ford's important book *The Dark Side of the Light Chasers*. Light chasing refers to attempts to whitewash shadow with a rampant idealistic, sweetness-and-light philosophy.

One of my former colleagues in California was fond of greeting others with a robust "Hey man, how are you . . . *good?*" His forced positivity and unwavering cheer left many of us quietly suspect. *It's all good* may reflect a heavenly truth, but it should not be used to obfuscate real-world dilemmas. There is wisdom in the old notion that those who are too heavenly minded are of no earthly good.

Peter Pan, a popular symbol of light chasing, had no shadow. Instead, he came equipped with wings and a relentless boyish idealism. His shadow, torn off and stashed in a drawer, later had to be carefully sewn back onto him. In more classic symbolism, Icarus suffered from his unchecked aspiration of flying to the sun. It makes sense that the closer we get to a source of light, the larger the shadow we will cast. And this is as true of the limelight, where celebrities who are thrown up the pop charts regularly come crashing down.

Light chasing has found its way into the contemporary practice of psychotherapy as well. Motivated by a desire for quick fixes, patients and professionals alike can get waylaid into a denial of darkness. This often leads to a technique-focused, feel-good approach that is tantamount to putting a pretty bandage on an unexamined wound. Even more alarming is the increasingly popular trend of prescribing psychiatric medication to repress and deny symptoms of our shadows.

Carl Jung taught that anything that takes a position will cast a shadow. This is true of any political, psychological, or personal positions we take. Living in a world of duality, we cannot help but take positions. Our essential personal or psychological shadows are cast by the fundamental positions we take. "Tell me who you are," said Stephen Levine, "and I'll tell you the name of your suffering" (Healing into Life and Death Workshop, Phoenix, 1990). Who we are, our persona or presentation in the world, is often antithetical to and compensatory for our shadows. *Persona,* the Greek word for "mask," is the root of our word for person.

In what is, perhaps, his most popular admonition, Jung reminds us in the opening of this chapter that imaginings of light will not support our enlightenment. Just as we have confused literal darkness with metaphoric darkness, we confuse literal light with spirituality. John Staudenmaier (1996), Jesuit priest and historian, points out that metaphors of "enlightenment" were not always associated with scientific objectivity, orderliness, and advancement. Likewise, metaphors of darkness were not always linked to disorder, irrationality, and fear. We have lost sight of the medieval wisdom that our fundamental effort to understand things is not always helped by clarity nor hurt by uncertainty.

When we fail to take responsibility for our shadows, we inevitably project them onto others and into the world. Then we shadowbox, engaging in protracted, self-righteous, and futile battles with our projections. In a brilliant essay on shadow in America, Jungian therapist Jeremy Abrams (1999) describes the modern collective manifestation of disowned shadow:

> The collective shadow—human evil in some malignant form—echoes back at us from virtually every

direction: it shouts from newsstand headlines; it squats in the X-rated neon pornography shops on the periphery of our cities; it wanders our streets, sleeping in doorways, homeless; it embezzles our life savings from the local savings and loan; it corrupts power-hungry politicians; it perverts our systems of justice; it drives our military arsenals toward the brink of insanity; it sells arms to mad leaders and gives the profits to reactionary insurgents; it pours pollution through hidden pipes into our rivers and oceans and poisons our food with invisible pesticides; it steals the cash in leveraged buyouts and insider trading, and threatens our health with defective technology and false promises, with medical claims and disastrous side-effects.

It is common practice in our world to define ourselves in terms of who we are not—in terms of shadow projections. Some people do not know who they are unless they have an enemy. "I'm going to do something terrible to you," said Soviet president Mikhail Gorbachev to U.S. president Ronald Reagan. It was the era of perestroika, the time associated with the dissolution of the Soviet Union. "I'm going to take away your enemy."

Ultimately, the question is not whether we will contend directly with our shadow issues or not. It is simply about how we will do so. Understanding shadow and truly committing to shadow work allow us to avert the problems of opportunistic emergence. We must learn to take back the night and its darkness.

The Nature of Shadow

Shadow and its characteristic darkness has long been associated with notions of evil. Darkness is a common synonym for evil. Hell, of course, is located deep underground, and beneath its searing flames, it is perpetually frozen and utterly dark. We know the devil as the Prince of Darkness. Familiar to us all, he sports hooves, horns, and a goatee, suggesting his base, animal nature.

In contrast, darkness has also been associated with spiritual beginnings. Like a number of others, the biblical account of creation begins with darkness. The Hebrew notion of *Ein Soff*, or endlessness, refers to the infinite sea of darkness from which light and all creation emerges. From the Jewish perspective, the new day does not start with dawn but with dusk and darkness.

The implication here is that darkness holds invisible seeds of light that can transform and heal us and our world. Darkness sensitizes us to more subtle forms of light. The human eye is capable of detecting a single photon, the smallest measurable unit of light, but it can only do so in absolute darkness.

In thinking back to my mother's experience in concentration camp, I believe her encounter with genuine evil by day allowed her to clearly distinguish it from the literal darkness of night. Jung warned of the dangers in confusing shadow or the appearance of darkness with evil. In one of his less popular positions, he emphasized that it was not the shadow, per se, but the ego that was evil. In essence, shadow contains both darkness and light.

As we emerge from night, our shadows grow shorter through morning, from dawn until noon. At high noon, when light is directly overhead, at the height of our waking day, we appear not to have a shadow. In actuality, we are standing on it. And in anticipation of the return of night, our shadows grow longer through the afternoon to disappear again at dusk, at which time they begin to swallow us. At night, our hemisphere is caught in the planet's shadow. Kabbalistic tradition teaches that the period between 6 p.m. and midnight is the most psychologically challenging part of the day. It is both literally and figuratively a time of increasing darkness.

Throughout most of history, dusk and darkening were not an option but an imperative. Small fires, candles, lanterns, and other early sources of nighttime light provided only minimal illumination compared to today's light bulb. A single 100-watt bulb, for example, concentrates the light of about 100 candles, allowing the average person today to easily surpass the illuminating ability of even the most privileged people of prior eras. For most of us today, wilderness camping experiences are as close as we can come to approximating how our ancestors may have routinely experienced dusk.

I have fond memories of such childhood campouts. In fact, what has remained most vivid for me are recollections of the arrival of dusk and the descent of darkness. As dusk approached, we scurried to wind down but also wound down our scurrying. With diminishing light, the outer world quieted, cooled, and softened, magically transforming before our very eyes. We obeyed this natural imperative to slow down much better than we might have obeyed our parents' request to do the same. As it grew darker, we were drawn to our campsite, gathering around a small fire for our evening meal. After dinner we huddled tightly to protect ourselves from the encroaching darkness. And inspired by the darkening and shadowy hills and trees all around, we told stories, stories that matched the ambient mood—ghost stories.

To date, little systematic historical or cross-cultural study has been completed of sleep practices in general and of social practices around dusk in particular. Naturalistic observations, however, suggest that with the advent of darkness, people probably behaved much like we did on camping trips. They would slow down, gather together around a source of low light, and probably process their fears and anxieties. I believe that this reflects an archetypal instinct to address shadow issues in a social context as night approaches. It is a way of washing away accumulated fears, a spiritual cleansing of the psyche in preparation for bed and the nightly journey into sleep and dreams.

Despite a growing interest in the psychology of shadow, little attention has been paid to the obvious relationship of shadow to literal darkness—to dusk and night. I believe that nighttime is an ideal medium for addressing and managing shadow issues.

In modern life, the most common source of light people are likely to gather around in the evening is a television set. And here we are more apt to discuss the evening news or the highlights of a sitcom than personal issues. Excessive nighttime television is a testament to our dependence on day. In lieu of honest contact with night, we remain glued to electronically reconstituted images of day.

My writing was just interrupted by a noise from the other side of the house. I am here alone—or at least I think I am. It's night, plenty dark out. Generally, I am not a person who is afraid *of the dark*. But I just noticed again how easy it is for my fear to come up *in the dark*. Darkness provides an open arena for whatever shadowy thoughts and feelings may be lurking behind day—what we might have hidden in the light.

It's embarrassing to admit, but I'm wondering if it could be a terrorist with a portable nuclear device . . . or something. I don't know. So . . . I check. And . . . there's nothing there. Probably a neighbor, or maybe that curious orange tabby that has been trying to break into my house. I take the opportunity to grab that last crumbling slice of apple pie from the refrigerator as I pass through the kitchen. Fear tends to zap one's energy. Food helps.

Oh, no. I think I hear it again—and, I'm out of pie.

Shadow Work

> *Wave on wave of life*
> *Like the great wide oceans roll*
> *Haunting hands of memory*
> *Pluck silver strands of soul*
> *The damage and the dying done*
> *The clarity of light*
> *Gentle bows and glasses raised*
> *To the charity of night*
>
> THE CHARITY OF NIGHT, 1996

As Bruce Cockburn suggests in these lyrics, there is a charity of night. We find diamonds in coal. Jung taught that our shadows conceal creative, healing, and good and precious things. Just as the day starts with night and the universe is created out of darkness, creative and good things can emerge from our shadows.

Jung defined shadow as "the thing one has no wish to be" (as quoted in Abrams 1999). Shadow work, then, is about carefully sifting through and coming to terms with all that we have no wish to be. We enter a dialogue with our shadow figures as Jesus did with the demons he encountered, as Marie did with her nightmarish black stallion, and as the Dalai Lama does with his enemies. We carefully sift through the qualities, values, and abilities of our shadow figures. Without becoming or succumbing to our shadows, we develop a conscious relationship with them. We take what we need and we leave the rest.

"Thus, the challenge," says Jeremy Abrams (1999), ". . . is not to defeat the Devil within, but to confront it and to integrate its powers and strengths into the Self. . . . Such a confrontation is necessary if we are to become truly human; to be complete, all parts of the psyche must be accepted." In the Gnostic Gospel of Thomas, such a confrontation is encouraged: "If you bring forth what is within you, what you bring forth will save you. If you fail to bring forth what is within you, what you fail to bring forth will destroy you."

In *Care of the Soul*, Thomas Moore bluntly summarizes the challenge of shadow work:

> The shadow is a frightening reality. Anyone who talks glibly about integrating the shadow, as if you could chum up to the shadow the way you learn a foreign language, doesn't know the darkness that always qualifies shadow. (1992, 133)

Integrating our shadow may well be the most challenging work we do as humans, taking us to depths that are incomprehensible. Most of us are familiar with the plight of Job, who offers a bleak description of his archetypal shadow experience. "I go to the place of no return, to the land of gloom and deep shadow, to the land of deepest night, of deep shadow and disorder, where even the light is like darkness." *Even the light is darkness.* There is a gloom that is unspeakable, an impenetrable darkness, a place of no return.

A Christian conceptualization of shadow work was outlined in the writings of the great mystic Saint John of the Cross. He believed that achieving spiritual freedom required a descent into the depths of confusion, loss, and despair, traversing the *dark night of the soul.* Saint John defined the dark night of the soul as an extended journey of emptying the self to create space for the divine. "If a man wishes to be sure of the road he treads on," he wrote, "he must close his eyes and walk in the dark."

Hugh Prather points out that Jesus encountered demons on three separate occasions. If we expect Jesus to shun, repel, or destroy them, we are surprised at his response. Instead, Jesus gently confronts these dark figures, engaging them in conversation. He asks their names, invites them to speak their minds, and he listens. This outstanding teaching about developing a conscious relationship with shadow demonstrates the value of courageous confrontation. Since much of the force of shadow is derived from intense fear born of ambiguity, engaging our shadows brings clarification, and the demons are peacefully disempowered.

We saw a similar process reflected in Marie's encounter with her shadowy black stallion. As she courageously gave this animal a voice and listened to its story, she recognized important qualities that she had disowned. With a clearer understanding of the horse and its intentions, her fear diminished and her sense of self expanded to reclaim these disowned qualities.

Not too long after my experience at the spiritual retreat discussed at the opening of this chapter, I was introduced to an ancient Tibetan Buddhist practice called *Tonglen.* Over recent decades, Tibetans have undergone immense hardship and suffering—a protracted encounter with a real world manifestation of shadow and darkness. Their survival is due in large part to a philosophy of compassion, a philosophy that also informs the practice of Tonglen.

Tonglen refers to a set of meditative breathing practices that serve as an ideal model and technique for shadow work. In one respect, Tonglen is antithetical to our common Pollyanna approach. In contrast to breathing in sweetness and light and breathing out darkness and shadow, Tonglen actually calls for the inhalation of negativity and the exhalation of goodness. I will review a basic Tonglen exercise in the practices section at the end of this chapter.

Tonglen opens our hearts and minds to darkness, symbolically receiving it and spiritually transforming it. The practice encourages a compassionate confrontation with all adversity, with darkness and shadow. Through visualization, images associated with darkness and shadow are inhaled. Within our chest, they are then reconfigured, discharged, and transformed. We literally inspire darkness and express healing light back into the world. The practice of Tonglen strengthens our psyches by reinforcing a sense of our profound capacity to transform darkness into light.

Shadow work is not simply about periodic meditative practices; it is about developing an enduring relationship with the darkness in our lives. Regular shadow work practices train us to remain open to the varying expressions of darkness we encounter in everyday life. When they are at our door, we metaphorically invite them in.

When Newman, also referred to as "the embodiment of evil," appeared at Jerry Seinfeld's door, he was allowed in. Ambivalent as Seinfeld was about this dark, greedy, deceptive, and all-around disagreeable character, he let him in. As crazy as Kramer was, he let him in, too. As hysterical as Elaine could be, she got in. And as narcissistic as George was, he also always was invited in.

I am not suggesting we literally allow the Newmans of the world into our living space, only into our hearts. We develop a relationship with shadow issues by allowing them into our psychological space.

I am, admittedly, a bit sheepish about including a reference to a television show about nothing in a chapter that addresses the critical human challenge of shadow. But how we posture toward the people close to us, our inevitable daily hassles, our own neuroses, and the ebb and flow of psychological duskiness is an important aspect of shadow work. These are precisely the kinds of challenges that appear most frequently in the course of our everyday lives.

Over the course of their TV friendships, Jerry Seinfeld not only invited his strange friends into his apartment but also admitted some of their qualities into his life. Seinfeld's appeal was in his receptivity, even, at times, to the absurd. Sometimes he took on qualities of his friends—even of his archenemy, Newman. Seinfeld breathed them into his space, shortcomings and all, and then breathed out lightheartedness.

Shadow Work Practices

Shadow work is not simple, nor is it easy, but it is essential if we are committed to healing night. The following exercises are offered to help you become more sensitive to the role of shadow in your sleep, dreaming, and waking.

Reel in Shadow Projections

Let yourself be more sensitive to the presence of shadow in your life. Be cognizant of your thoughts about common hosts of projections like politicians and car salesmen. Also, be cognizant of shadow issues triggered by the people closest to you—your coworkers, friends, partner, and family members.

Keep a running list of all the negative qualities of people you react to, including public figures. Are they too sweet or selfish, too rich or poor, too deceptive or outspoken? Study the charged judgments you may have. Do some of these reflect characteristics you deny in yourself? Allow yourself to sift through these judgments in search of any underlying positive features. Do some of your judgments contain kernels of qualities you actually need or want more of in your life?

Practice Tonglen

The basic Tonglen practice can be applied in a formal, organized manner or more loosely adapted to virtually any challenging situation or setting. Essentially, Tonglen is about opening one's heart and mind to specific shadowy images in any form—people, places, events, heavy emotions, or any other challenging experiences.

To practice Tonglen, begin by taking a moment to relax, become as physically comfortable and psychologically centered as you can. As you inhale, imagine you are drawing in whatever specific shadowy image or issue you want to heal. Breathe it into yourself slowly and deeply, including whatever difficult or painful emotions may be associated with it. Then, slowly exhale a vision of healing, relief, compassion, freedom, and peace. Continue this process for a few moments or for as long as is comfortable. Try repeating this practice on a regular basis. Since it is portable and requires no equipment or special setting, try using it during moments of adversity throughout the day.

Dusky Night of the Soul

We have seen that the opportunistic emergence of anxieties and shadow issues can interfere with our natural relationship with night and sleep. Our issues emerge opportunistically only when we do not give them due consideration at more appropriate times. This is particularly true during crisis periods of our lives, times of strong shadow emergence.

Keep in mind that evening is an ideal time for shadow work. Dusk naturally promotes our "letting go" practices. Consider journaling about your shadow issues during dusk simulation. Begin a regular practice of processing the day, including its shadowy experiences, with your partner or family members. In this way, you can resolve some of your nightmares before you get into bed.

⌣

Healing night and night consciousness requires that we overcome our primal fear of darkness. Some things are seen more clearly in the dark. Some things can be seen only in the dark. The essential lesson of shadow work is that even darkness contains light. It is not the ordinary, fluctuating light of this world but the steady, spiritual illumination of a larger sphere. It is a kind of light that can best be experienced away from the distractions of day, in the quiet of night.

∼9

Imagination:
The Waking Dream

*They who dream by day are cognizant of many things
that escape those who dream only by night.*

—EDGAR ALLAN POE

SOME YEARS AGO I had the distinct privilege of studying with
James, an unusual hybrid of psychotherapist and shaman, an expert in Jungian psychology who was equally comfortable in the
ethereal world of the dream. Early in my studies with James, I
enrolled in his Imaginal Seminar, a ten-week intensive course on
dreams and the world of imagination.

Participants in this course were asked to carefully attend to and
thoroughly journal their nightly dreams. I managed to train myself
to awaken repeatedly throughout the night to record the details of
my dreams. I was surprised at how quickly the pages of my dream
journal filled up with a range of rich and mysterious experiences.
James also asked us to keep a diary, a journal of our waking experiences. Curiously, however, he specifically asked us to reflect on and
record our waking experiences *as if they were dreams.*

"What?" a number of us asked in unison. James just smiled.

Over the coming weeks James's instructions crystallized. Usually, keeping a diary or journal entails recording and reflecting on
day-to-day, ordinary life experiences. We might enter descriptions
of what we did that day, the people we encountered, the feelings
we had, and our thoughts about all of these. A diary of this sort

usually consists of a running account of our daily lives with some personal commentary and, possibly, some evaluation. Typically we fail to recognize that we selectively attend only to those aspects of our daily lives that our culture and ego deem relevant.

We fail to notice so many things because we consider them incidental, irrelevant, or peripheral to our lives. We fail to notice clouds morphing into mythic animals, the surprisingly familiar face in a crowd of total strangers, the curious appearance of feathers and stones strewn along our hurried path, and the peculiar coincidences that seem to outnumber the possibility of probability. We also fail to notice the musings of our imagination that accompany such experiences. These things call to us with a whisper that remains oddly audible despite the ruckus of our driven lives.

If we were recounting a nighttime dream, these are precisely the kinds of images that would leap out at us. Dream images are usually presumed to have inherent symbolic value or meaning. Because we instinctively expect and, therefore, seek meaning in a dream, we take notice of these seemingly incidental experiences. And because we do not expect to find this same kind of meaning in waking life, we simply fail to notice it. Ordinary waking life, in contrast to dream consciousness, is more concerned with function and productivity than with image and meaning. It is, by design, mundane.

As I recorded my daily life experiences as if they were a dream, the symbolic undercurrent of seemingly incidental experiences became increasingly evident. I grew curious about the shapes of clouds, the faces of strangers, feathers and stones. I became more sensitive to "ordinary things"—my own thoughts, feelings, and, especially, imaginings. Although nothing in my world changed, virtually everything began to take on more depth, meaning, and mystery. Ordinary relevance became less relevant. Almost overnight, I also began noticing more coincidences and became enamored with the notion of synchronicity. Just as I was speaking to a friend about this, my son called with a question. He had just bought an album called *Synchronicity* and wondered what it meant. With admission of the symbolic and the imaginal, life became so much richer.

After a few weeks of recording my nightly dreams alongside of my daily life as a dream, I began experiencing a disturbing phenomenon. Because my waking and dream lives were no longer sharply segregated, I found myself confusing reality with the fantasy of the imaginal. The memories of my nightly and waking dreams were melding with those of my waking experiences. Images from a dream the night before, for example, felt as real and vivid as the events of my waking day. It was as if the fantasy world of dreaming had become as immediate, significant, and compelling as the real world of waking. Although I functioned perfectly well, I sometimes confused memories of actual waking life events with those of dream events.

One does not have to be a psychologist to know that confusing fantasy with reality in this way can be symptomatic of a serious mental disorder. I nervously arranged a meeting with James to share my concerns.

"James," I said, "my mind is really mixing stuff up here. There are moments when I'm having trouble just distinguishing the real, waking world from my dream world. It's like the two are just blending into one big world." James nodded with empathy as he smiled one of his impossibly large and reassuring smiles. He put his hand on my shoulder and whispered, "Great."

The Waking Dream

We dream all the time. There is compelling biological, psychological, and spiritual evidence suggesting that ongoing dreamlike experiences are woven throughout the entire day. Like stars, dreams appear to come out only at night. In actuality, they are there all the time. And like the daytime sky, our ordinary waking consciousness casts an illusory canopy overhead that obscures our view of a much bigger world. It is like a dropped ceiling, offering some sense of containment and security, but only at the dear cost of significantly constrained consciousness.

As we saw, the rest phases of our basic rest and activity cycles are associated with a shift into a more relaxed, diffused, and imaginal consciousness. This is a natural portal to the waking dream, a regular eclipse of our waking consciousness in which the mind's sky opens, offering a glimpse of the infinite. Although this experience may be hazy and overexposed in comparison to our nighttime REM dreams, it is nonetheless a gracious reminder of that bigger world.

The waking dream is *a sacred way of perceiving*. It is not an alternative to ordinary waking consciousness but an enhancement of it. The waking dream is not about seeing beyond our ordinary lives to some dreamy, ethereal vision. It is about seeing our ordinary lives anew in a more dreamlike and ethereal way. It is a slower and more mindful way of perceiving that senses a bashful intelligence quivering behind all things.

Intentionally opening to the waking dream brings the promise of reenchanting lives deeply entrenched in the mundane. Because it expands our frame of reference, the waking dream opens a grand vista to the play of synchronicity. It can help us restore our lost sense of the numinous, the spirituality of everyday life—what Carl Jung called the *symbolic view of life*. As a way of perceiving, the waking dream sees through the mundane to the sacred. "The miracle is not to walk on water," teaches Thich Nhat Hanh, "the miracle is to walk on land" (2001, 23).

Since the start of time, human beings have demonstrated an almost universal interest and reverence for the important place of imagination and the waking dream in daily life. From Christian mystical practices to Celtic and earth-based traditions, from indigenous cultures like the Australian Aboriginals and Native Americans to Eastern Hindu and Buddhist techniques, from the Greeks to the Chinese, and from the Sufis to the Kabbalists—all developed sacred practices for relating to the waking dream. The waking dream has also been a powerful medium of many healing practices ranging from depth psychology to various forms of shamanism.

Despite its wondrous potential, like the night dream, the waking dream is largely disregarded, and waking dream work has nearly been lost in our modern world. As a superbly personal and subjective experience, the waking dream cannot thrive in a culture that places such a heavy premium on objective experience. The individual imagination has been displaced by collective social structures that serve our driven lifestyles. Hungry for the deeply personal, natural dream, we are offered an artificial substitute in the form of entertainment.

Industrial culture has reduced imagination to a real-world commodity that can be mass produced, purchased, and consumed. Imagination has been abducted from its natural home in our hearts and is being held captive in theme parks, virtual reality games, movies, and television shows. Even the great big imagination of a really small child cannot compete with men in giant mouse suits. Adults are an easier target still, succumbing quickly to a glass of cheap wine and "reality" TV.

I have no argument with most forms of entertainment, per se. But these are no substitute for imagination. DreamWorks cannot legitimately replace dream work. Observing the artistic expression of others can certainly be inspirational and motivating, but it is about as nourishing as watching someone else eat. Though we can certainly derive pleasure in observing those we care about take nourishment, we still need our own. The entertainment industry's spiritual sleight of hand has drawn our vital energies away from the heart, from ourselves, from our personal dreams. We spend significantly more time attending to television than we do to our own inner vision. We watch movies about others' lives rather than moving watchfully through our own. And we remain seriously undernourished, starved for the spiritual sustenance of an expansive dream awareness.

Earlier I suggested that nighttime dream deprivation could leave us pathologically dreamy by day. I believe that REM pressure resulting from the loss of night dreams seeps back into our daytime consciousness at both individual and collective levels. The symptoms of fatigue, scattered attention, fuzzy mindedness, the inability to concentrate may be compensatory reactions that draw us back toward dismissed dreamy experiences. At a collective level, it is interesting to consider the possible connection between daytime dream rebound and the symptoms of certain sleep disorders.

Narcolepsy and REM behavior disorder (RBD) are two sleep disorders in which the boundary between dreaming and waking becomes excessively permeable. In both of these conditions, specific features of night dreaming intrude into waking. Narcolepsy is not, as is commonly believed, a disorder characterized by "sleep attacks." Although it is associated with excessive daytime sleepiness, it is more accurately characterized by *cataplexy,* the spontaneous intrusion of sleep paralysis into waking consciousness. Likewise, RBD, characterized by the failure of sleep paralysis, results in an unexpected breakthrough of nighttime dream activity into the waking world. To varying degrees, people with RBD involuntarily act out their dreams as they are happening. Beyond the medical and psychological complexities of these conditions, narcolepsy and RBD may well be further spiritual symptoms of our collective dream deprivation.

The waking dream broadens our frame of perception, allowing us to witness a deeper order behind all things—behind clouds, strangers, feathers, and stones. And behind earthquakes, wars, psychopaths, and roaches. Although it opens us to lovely and joyous perceptions, the waking dream is not about the contemporary spirituality of sweetness and light. It also insists that we remain open to dusk and darkness, to night, nightmares, and shadow. Unfortunately, this offends our sanitized spiritual sensibilities and may be one of the main reasons we shun the waking dream and the world of imagination.

Numinosity: A Symbolic View of Daily Life

The waking dream calls for a way of being that Jung referred to as the *symbolic view of life.* It is a perceptual style that wholeheartedly invites imagination and dreamlike experiences into waking life. It is a lucid way of seeing because it presumes that all things have symbolic value or meaning. And because value and meaning are personal, subjective, and experiential, it eases our pathological extraversion and restores the role of inner experience to our spirituality.

A common spiritual principle suggests that motivation determines perception, and perception determines the world we live in.

We generally proceed through daily life with perceptions that are defined and framed by our intentions. What we want, our motivation or intention, determines how we look at the world and, consequently, what we see. Intention casts a basic frame around our perceptions. And for many of us today, it is a driven, industrious frame.

Industrial culture imbues a ubiquitous and subtle intention toward utility into most everything we do. We unconsciously look for and pay attention to things that are meaningful in terms of this standard. Our industrious intentions result in a kind of pervasive work ethic that filters most experience through the question, *how might I use this?* Even when we are away from formal work, we are often on the make. We might step up the pace of an after-dinner stroll to squeeze some aerobic benefit out of it, sleep becomes part of our health maintenance program, and even friends secretly function as part of our business network. This mentality may be the subtlest form of the substance abuse–related notion of "using," in which some ulterior motive overrides so many of our actions.

A symbolic view of life asks that we release our extraverted, industrious intention—that we stop persistently looking at the world with an eye for its utility. If we are willing to do so, we temporarily unframe our lives, our intentions, and perceptions. We restore a natural, innocent, and childlike sense of mystery and numinosity to our world. The waking dream is a way of perceiving that is driven less by ordinary intention and more by valuing the image itself, by a pure form of imagination. If waking intention is associated with the maxim "use it or lose it," the waking dream operates on the premise of "use it and you lose it."

To the ordinary mind, that feather on the sidewalk is little more than litter; it has no utility. Through the eyes of the waking dream, the image of this feather instantly reverberates with endless associations on themes of wings, sky, and aspiration. In contrast to industrious intent, which is concerned with utility, the waking dream is inherently concerned with the symbolic *image*, with the practice of experiencing and understanding that image, with intentional imagination.

The image was once a sacred notion associated with the creative process of imaging or representing spirit in the world of matter. The earth was created in the image of the heavens. We were imaged or imagined by the divine, made in the image of God. And because we are imbued with characteristics of divine creativity, we inherited this capacity for imagination, for the symbolic view of the world. Many sacred traditions emphasize the fundamental spiritual practice of tracing the symbolic image back to its ultimate source.

André Malraux wrote, in *Man's Fate:*

> The world is like the characters of our [Chinese] writing. What the symbol is to the flower, the flower itself . . . is to something. To go from the symbol to the thing symbolized is to explore the depth and meaning of the world, it is to seek God. (As quoted in Watkins 1976, 1)

Proceeding from the symbol to the thing symbolized helps realign us with the spiritual tenet of *as it is above so is it below.* This is the essential method of spiritual dream work.

Images in dreams often transform before our eyes. In fact, this sort of morphing (from Morpheus) seems to be one of the defining characteristics of dreaming. Animals turn into people. People become other people. And structures morph in a thousand ways. We see a similar transformation of images in the waking dream. Such transformations reveal the meaning held in the image. While we dream, we are experiencing the symbolic view of life—we innocently witness the symbolic value of images. This is true because we do not usually carry industrial strength intentions into our dreams.

Waking dreaming should not be confused with the spacey, escapist meanderings of a daydream. Although both involve imagination, their intentions are markedly different. In a daydream, our focus drifts away from the immediate world with some intention of escaping it. Even when the subject of the daydream may be something of value and desirable, it is much more a mindless escape than a conscious quest.

In contrast, the waking dream is intentionally unintentional. Its purpose is simple receptivity to spiritual experience and exploration of what is. How we relate to this nonmaterial world of images, this waking dreamscape, is a clear reflection of our basic posture toward our spirituality.

The waking dream is an essentially spiritual, though not necessarily ordinary or natural, way of seeing. Medieval alchemists described the waking dream as an *opus contra naturum,* a process in opposition to our ordinary nature. Ordinarily, perception involves attention and focus on immediate matters—the world of matter all around us. From a survival perspective, it makes sense that we are programmed to attend to the exigencies of this world. The very word *matter,* which refers to the material world, has come to denote value—what *matters.* Our perception is firmly and unconsciously fixed upon and grounded in the world of matter. Like a modern camera, the process of perception automatically focuses on what matters, on the material world. And we then trace our experiences—our sensations, thoughts, feelings, and intuitions back down to their material associations.

Although it is what matter represents, in one sense, the image is the opposite of matter. And the imaginal realm, as it has been called, can be seen as the antithesis of the material world. The waking dream, then, is a way of perceiving that traces our experiences *backward,* away from "what matters" and toward an extrasensory world. The waking dream blurs our ordinary vision as it calls our attention to the spiritual realm. Instead of grounding, it untethers us. Instead of comforting us with familiarities, it unsettles us with possibilities. It is a way of looking up, a way of perceiving the spiritual atmosphere surrounding and sustaining the world of matter.

The Half Dream

The waking dream may be more readily accessed at the edges of sleep. Many people report spontaneous experiences of being in a half-dream, half-waking state as they are falling asleep or waking up. Known as *hypnagogic hallucinations,* these hybrid, half-dream experiences have been widely reported across cultures and time. They are of interest to sleep scientists primarily because they are frequently, but certainly not exclusively, associated with narcolepsy.

I have spoken with many people (most without narcoleptic symptoms) over the years who eventually acknowledged having such half-dream experiences, but only after they felt psychologically safe. They had refrained from openly discussing them with others because the experiences were so strange, extraordinary, and even otherworldly. As well as fearing being misunderstood or getting diagnosed with a mental disorder, I believe at some level, many recognized that they had ventured into potentially sacred territory. But they had no viable frame of reference for making sense of their experiences.

Alan was a doctor who held back for some years before he allowed himself to talk about his first half dream:

> Although I was in bed with my eyes closed, I was
> fully awake and could actually look around and
> see my bedroom as I had left it the night before.
> My body felt kind of eerie, very heavy and light
> at the same time. It wasn't a bad feeling, though
> it was unusual and unsettling. My bedroom door
> was open and I could see a large Native American
> man dressed in a black Western outfit and hat just
> casually stroll in. Somehow, I knew he was looking
> for his wife who was already in the room. Somehow,
> I also knew he was a medicine man even though I
> didn't really understand what that meant. And de-
> spite my sense that he was not dangerous, I became
> very frightened about peering into this other awe-
> some world.

The half dream can trigger immense fear, particularly when one is unfamiliar with the experience and it contains mysterious or shadowy images. As a mix of the fantastic imagery and REM paralysis of nighttime dreaming and the strong sense of reality associated with waking, the half dream can feel extremely intense—even more real than ordinary waking. Obtaining a frame of reference for understanding the half dream can help diminish the fear it commonly elicits. Either scientific or spiritual frames of reference can work, though each opens and closes different doors. Conventional sleep medicine understands the half dream in terms of neurophysiological glitches. It further labels these experiences as "hallucinations," placing an unnecessary pathological spin on them.

Not all half dreams are frightening. Suzanne, a forty-five-year-old software engineer, experienced half dreams, or what she referred to as "dreamtime," throughout much of her life. She came to terms with the fact that they were a kind of family legacy, not at all pathological, and potentially enjoyable.

> While I love dreamtime and am very lucky (they are generally pleasant), it can be disturbing to wake up with people in the room with you—I've learned to live with it and it isn't scary—they are generally just annoying now. My husband has noticed that I sleep with my eyes open a lot—and my son does it as well and that probably is part of it—at some point, the room objects invade my dreams and vice versa. Fortunately, I've only had two live nightmares (my whole life) so I can't complain. Once I woke up to a room full of beautiful hummingbirds flying all over—so sometimes it's actually a great pleasure— well, at least to me. I've stopped waking up my husband to say, "Can you see . . ."

Permeability between the world of waking and that of dreaming is valued and actively pursued in many traditional approaches to healing and spirituality. *Shamanism* is a general term applied to special healing and spiritual practices that operate through the medium of the waking dream. Shamans, who are present in diverse cultures around the world, usually undergo extensive and challenging training to acquire their special skills. In recent years, various shamanic practices have made their way into the Western world and can be useful tools for understanding the connection between our dream lives and the waking world. While I acknowledge narcolepsy's medical complexities, I prefer to think of it as a form of reluctant shamanism.

Odd as it may seem from a conventional medical perspective, the Program in Integrative Medicine at the University of Arizona includes a shamanic practitioner among its multidisciplinary team of preceptors. I believe waking dream work will play an increasingly important role in the future of medicine and psychotherapy.

Many people have explored personal approaches to accessing the waking dream. A half century before the discovery of REM sleep, Salvador Dalí experimented with methods of accessing his dreams while awake. He found that depriving himself of sleep for significant periods increased the intensity and volume of his dreams. (Something sleep science has since confirmed.) Dalí also stumbled upon a curious strategy to enhance his creative process. After preparing his easel and palette to paint, he reclined in a soft chair, holding a metal kitchen utensil in his hand suspended over a tin plate on the floor. Dalí would then allow himself to drift off to sleep. When he entered REM sleep he would, of course, lose muscle tone, and his hand would relax and open, dropping the utensil onto the metal plate to wake him up. In this way, Dalí could intentionally awaken within dream states to enter a waking dreamlike consciousness and paint.

Accessing the Waking Dream

We can also readily access the waking dream directly from waking states. In my work with dreams over three decades, I have observed a number of essential characteristics pertinent to the dreaming processes. Independent of dream content, most dreams seem to occur within a predictable framework, defined by specific *dream coordinates*. These are less about the characteristics of dreams themselves and more about the ways in which we experience them. If dreams were movies, dream coordinates would be about the structure of the theater.

Dream coordinates include *dream time, dream space, dream self,* and *dream spirit. Dream time* is about the tempo of our perception. It is a kind of slow-motion, present-moment way of seeing. In lieu of common spatial perceptual frames, *dream space* is about an expansive, permeable, unframed way of seeing. From within dream space and dream time, one's sense of a *dream self* can emerge and morph freely beyond the bounds of what we know to be possible. And throughout all of this, we witness the essential and ineffable *dream spirit* of numinosity. Although we can segregate our discussion of these dream coordinates, in actuality, they are interdependent, even interlocked.

Dream coordinates describe the psychological posture we instinctively assume while we dream. In a sense, they define the dreamer. Intentionally assuming this posture during waking can help us consciously access the waking dream.

Dream Time

One's sense of time in a dream can be remarkably malleable, though we seem to experience most dreams in the present moment. Rarely are we preoccupied with the past or future; the present moment is much too poignant. And because dreams happen in the *now*, the movement in dreams takes on a slow-motion quality. Dream time discourages racing or speeding, even when we might want to. Whether I am sitting still or running for my life, most dream experiences are characterized by a peculiar slowness. Independent of the nature of the dream, dream time itself is generally more relaxed than waking time.

Dream Space

Around its edges, dream space is highly permeable, if not completely unframed. It reveals a bigger picture, a much bigger world.

Dream space does not so much open a new path as it unveils a surprising and expansive panorama. All things become more richly contextualized. The feather on the sidewalk is not just a feather; it is an integral and accessible element of this new and mysterious panorama.

The relaxed nature of dream time is associated with an expanded perceptual field. We experience more when we slow down. In a sense, our gaze relaxes and opens like a wide-angle lens. Studies show that our perceptual field can expand dramatically in dreams. We notice more of the periphery and context of what we are experiencing. We know, for example, that it is certainly possible to be in a building and simultaneously observe it from the outside. (This, of course, is not permitted in ordinary waking consciousness.)

Dream Self

Who I am in a dream is usually more fluid than my sense of self in waking. I can be an active player in my dream, immersed fully in its drama and emotion. Or I may scarcely be present in the action of the dream, sitting back and experiencing it as an observer. Often, there is a mix of the two: I can be both in and observing my experience simultaneously.

My dream self is generally not as narrowly defined by my ego, the limiting perceptual sets of my waking life. Since my expanded self does not know or believe that it cannot fly, for example, it can. The dream self can be significantly more open and malleable than the waking self. Just as Marie discovered that she was the horse in her nightmare, the "I" figure in our dreams is capable of an expanded identification with all aspects of the dream. I am, for example, myself walking down the street. And I am the street.

Dream Spirit

Dreams are the natural home of all that is numinous. From the Greek *numen,* which suggests the endorsement of the gods, *numinosity* refers to reflections of a divine presence in all things. Flowing in dream time through dream space, our dream self can witness life unveiled, laden with mystery and meaning. We see in a symbolical way in our dreams.

This dream spirit is awareness expanded to accommodate a subtle but larger order living behind all things. Because it broadens our frame of perception, it allows us to see evidence of the divine in all beings, in clouds and rocks and, of course, even in that feather on the sidewalk. The dream spirit is innocent and fierce, ancient but fresh, mysterious, yet familiar, and it is, even in its darkest manifestations, potentially good.

These specific "dream coordinates" of dream time, dream space, dream self, and dream spirit are overlapping and interlocked. Although they can be applied and practiced independently, they will ultimately integrate and become second nature. But, maybe it is more accurate to think of them as our primary nature. I believe this is how we naturally looked upon the world as children. In that sense, the process is less one of learning and more about remembering.

The notion of remembrance is key to many spiritual approaches, including waking dream work. The Hindu Vedas state, "All of this struggle to learn, when all we really must do is remember." As a way of seeing, waking dreaming is a skill that can be practiced and learned, or more accurately, remembered. What is the essence of remembrance? In contrast to learning, in remembering we are aware that we already possess what we are seeking—it is simply about accessing it. Most of us know that when we have something on the "tip of the tongue," the key to recalling what we cannot remember is relaxation. I believe it is similar with spiritual remembering. Waking dreaming calls for a relaxed and faithful posture.

This relaxed, faithful posture is based on the presumption of meaning. As I suggested earlier, I believe it is more important to know that dreams are meaningful than it is to know precisely what they mean. The waking dream can be approached not only from a common *interpretation* perspective but also from this broader, *relation* perspective. Beyond the obvious benefit of discovering personal and transpersonal meaning associated with the waking dream is this deeper, though more subtle, value in establishing a relationship to the dream world.

Waking Dream Practices

The following exercises may help you access your waking dreams and encourage personal awareness of their presence and gifts.

Keep a Waking Dream Journal

Maintaining a waking dream journal is an excellent way to gently develop a relationship with the waking dream world. This is best done a few moments prior to bed. Begin with a relaxed frame of mind. Using the dream coordinates discussed above, recount your day as if it were a dream. You could review your day in terms of the sequence of events, keeping an eye open for images and symbols you ordinarily consider "mundane." As an alternative, you could recount your day in terms of specific emotional, spiritual, or other themes. Combine this process with regular dream journaling and you may notice common themes weaving through both your night and waking dreams.

Practice Active Imagination

Active imagination refers to a set of Jungian-based techniques for accessing the waking dream. These techniques are adaptive and can be used to elaborate on your understanding of a night dream or to explore the unconscious in a waking state. Basically, active imagination calls for a deep state of waking relaxation during which the mind is encouraged to express and observe dream consciousness. This requires holding a nonjudgmental and noninterpretive stance toward the images that arise. Remembering that this imaginative or dream process may occur at a symbolic level can help you suspend judgment, allowing the experience to unfold freely.

Active imagination can be done on your own, with the support of a friend, or in a professional setting with a counselor or therapist.

Usually such sessions take about ten to fifteen minutes and are journaled afterward.

Consider Sandplay

Sandplay refers to a powerful form of depth psychotherapy developed primarily by Carl Jung and his student Dora Kalf. It involves working with a specially trained therapist who utilizes a miniature sandbox and a collection of dozens of figurines. Sandplay involves selecting figurines (people, animals, as well as a wide array of other objects) and arranging them to form an image in the sandbox. This image is then explored with the therapist. Sandplay accesses the unconscious, according to Kalf, at a level beneath the place where dreams are formed. In this way it serves as a unique bridge between dreaming and waking.

Developed originally for children, sandplay has been widely used with adults around the world in recent decades. It is effective at safely accessing preverbal and other nonverbal experiences. As a form of therapy or self-exploration, it is less directive and more spiritually affirmative. In short, sandplay provides a metaphoric "MRI" of the soul. Sandplay has been used as an adjunct to addressing a wide range of emotional and physical disorders as well as in support of personal psychological and spiritual growth. I believe it is particularly useful in treating problems associated with dream loss, including depression and cancer.

Sandplay is one of the best ways I know to access the imaginal realm and the waking dream. Qualified sandplay practitioners can be located through local Friends of Jung organizations.

Explore the Waking Dream in Everyday Stories

Myths, fables, fairy tales, and similar stories are to culture what the dream is to the individual. We can learn much from the study of such stories that have withstood the challenge of time. Our lives today are part of an emerging story that, hopefully, will be told in future centuries. The waking dream perspective can help us understand our emerging story. Let yourself look at the sweep of local, national, and global current events as if they were a dream. Try using the dream coordinates to reframe the news into the emerging myth of our time.

A Note on Waking Dream Work

Waking dream work is not for everyone. Sometimes the boundary between waking and dreaming can be excessively and uncomfortably permeable. Personal traumatic experiences, severe abuse in childhood, emotional instability, and drug reactions can damage or tear the dream-wake boundary in some individuals. On the other hand, some people have used their accidental access to the waking dream to promote healing and spiritual growth. If you feel uncomfortable about waking dream matters, you would be wise to obtain qualified professional or spiritual guidance.

⌇

In time, with a growing regard for the dream, we come to feel at home in another place in consciousness, in imagination. It is a place where sacred traditions are born, where dream cultures live, where artists work, and where children play. As we proceed, the boundary between waking and dreaming—between reality and a broader reality—becomes increasingly permeable. Uncontained, the constricted outer world we believe to be real now pales in comparison. Like an airplane ascending through a low ceiling of thick cloud cover, we break through to a vast and clear sky. It is a distinctly familiar place. Always much bigger than we remembered, perhaps it is too majestic for us tolerate on a regular basis but certainly worth the try.

⌒ 10

Integrating Consciousness

Human consciousness has developed on the one planet where the lights that rule day and night are equal.

—ANDREW WEIL, M.D.

IN *THE WORLD AND OTHER PLACES*, British author Jeanette Winterson provides us with a glimpse into a future in which the value of sleep has continued to erode:

> Most of the jobs advertised these days insist on a non-sleeper. Sleeping is dirty, unhygienic, wasteful and disrespectful to others. All public spaces are designated 'Non-Sleeping' and even a quick nap on a park bench carries £50 fine. You can still sleep in your own home but all new beds are required by law to have a personal alarm clock built into the mattress. If you get caught on a bed-check with a dead alarm, that's another £50 fine. Three fines and you are disqualified from sleeping for a year.
>
> I don't have a new bed. When I invited my girlfriend to my flat for the first time, she had never seen a bed like mine.
>
> "Wow. Is that an antique?"
>
> "Do you like antiques?"
>
> "Well, they're so . . . old."
>
> "This is my bed. My one and only."

"What do you use it for?"

"I sleep in it."

"For special occasions?"

"Every night. Nine or ten hours every night."

"You mean every week."

I took her in my arms. Tonight, this night, tomorrow night, the nights in gentle stars with you, if you like, rolled and dark and quilted with stars. I asked her to sleep with me.

"You mean lie awake with you? Everybody wants to know if we're lying awake together."

"Sleeping together."

She was worried. Now she knew she was with a real heavy number.

"Nine or ten hours a night?"

I nodded, addicted, dumb, sleep-hooked, sleepy. (1998, 105–6)

As we have seen, sleeping, dreaming, and waking disorders are in large part symptomatic of our night blindness—our underlying fear of darkness and the ensuing suppression of night. Nyx has been in exile too long. The sun and moon have been segregated, like night and day, like night consciousness and waking. Yin is torn from yang, leaving our lives virtually devoid of true rest. Seduced by culture's call to incessant drive, we have lost our resonance with life's natural rhythms and sputter along with now faltering counterfeit energies. As far-fetched as the opening sleep science fiction vignette may seem, it appears to be the direction we are heading in.

Lying awake together.

The effective resolution to our sleep, dream, and waking dilemmas calls for healing our relationship with Nyx—as an expression of both rhythmic order and of night, darkness, and night consciousness. Beyond our personal efforts at becoming more nightminded—our various lucidity and shadow work practices—I believe it is essential that we simultaneously consider a rapprochement with Nyx at a larger collective, community, and cultural level.

Righting Our Rhythms

Recently a group of Stanford University physicians raised concern about the dramatic decline in the variation of our experience of the natural environment. More specifically, they hypothesized that our extensive daytime sheltering from natural light and nighttime use of artificial light have reduced the range of our biological functions by altering natural melatonin cycles and, thereby, contributing to systemic health dysfunctions. They further state that therapeutic strategies that undermine our need to adapt "may actually impair future ability to respond to biologic disequilibria" (Yun et al. 2005, 1). In conclusion, they call for "therapeutic and lifestyle approaches that expand, rather than reduce, the dynamic range of many biologic experiences" (Yun et al. 2005, 1).

As we have seen, with diminished exposure to the natural environment, to sunlight by day and darkness at night, the naturally robust peaks and valleys of our circadian rhythms are indeed flattening. We have been attempting to compensate with the escalating use of counterfeit energies and chemical brakes. In lieu of a relationship with our natural environment, we depend heavily on alcohol, sleeping pills, and sheer exhaustion to slow and stop us at night, and caffeine, sugar, hyperbolic information, and LAN to keep us buzzing throughout our protracted days.

Despite our attempts at compensation, our sleeping, dreaming, and waking disorders continue to worsen, leaving us craving even harder stuff. Recent years have witnessed a dramatic increase in the interest, development, and use of new, more sophisticated generations of sleeping and waking pills.

I have used the term *waking pills* to refer to two classes of prescription medications that are designed to mask our growing depletion and daze. These include stimulants, medications that maintain alertness, as well as the newer antidepressants, which combat low mood and energy states, especially fatigue. In essence, waking pills mask daytime sleepiness. I believe it makes more sense to address such sleepiness at its source rather than at its symptoms.

Waking pills produce a form of artificial waking. These are dead-horse beaters—unrelenting energizers that not only override our need for rest but attempt to make up for years of overcompensation with other counterfeit energies. The long half-lives of waking pills inadvertently extend aspects of waking consciousness into the night, interfering with the rhythm of night consciousness, with our sleep and dreams. Ultimately, they threaten to inflict even greater damage on our natural circadian rhythms.

Likewise, we have seen that sleeping pills can do more damage than good. As damning information about popular sleeping pills becomes more public, the pharmaceutical industry continues to develop newer versions that undermine our natural sleep in new ways. The public, however, continues to be duped by the seductive and often misleading sleeping pill advertisements. Full-page glossy magazine ads tout the safety and wondrous soporific powers of these drugs. Turn the page. *Read the small print.*

Excessive dependence on any sleep or waking medications damages our sense of rhythmicity—biologically, psychologically, and spiritually. Ultimately, these kinds of medications are based on a mechanistic model that expects the body and mind to operate like a machine. Waking and sleeping pills simply do not work in tandem with our natural rhythms. They are chemical overcompensations that continue to push and pull at us relentlessly through our days and nights. Metaphorically, we end up simultaneously riding the accelerator and brake, wearing down our bodies and minds.

These medications also damage our psychological and spiritual sense of self-efficacy—our belief in our own natural, inherent ability to be awake, sleep, and dream. And just as badly, they interfere with our natural surrender to night and sleep as well as our natural awakening into dawn and day. It is time for us to aspire to a much greater pharmacological sobriety. Even as a culture, we need to detox.

Our grandparents' advice to get plenty of sunshine by day and turn the lights off at night reflects an intuitive wisdom that would serve us well today. We need to become more sensitive to the natural rhythms of day and night. We would, in fact, benefit from becoming more ritualized, much more rhythmic in our dance with night and day consciousness.

Resuscitating Nyx

I have emphasized that night is the best sleep medicine. Unfortunately, the quality of our nights is being seriously compromised by global light pollution, a lack of personal connection with the atmosphere of night, and the impact of chronic melatonin suppression. I believe we face a growing urgency to reinstate night into our lives, to resuscitate Nyx. To do so we must find ways to deluminate night, reestablish a personal relationship with the night sky, and carefully consider compensating for our chronic darkness deficiency with melatonin supplementation.

Like many of its citizens, our planet sleeps with too many lights on. Healing our relationship with Nyx is hampered by the simple fact that in most urban communities, she is barred from being fully present by light pollution.

Despite the fact that there is little rational basis for this excessive LAN, we beam immense amounts of light into the night, around our cities, into our neighbors' yards, and up into space. Just as many of us mindlessly turn lights on all over and around our homes at night, we do the same in the world around us. The International Dark Sky Association points out that most outdoor nighttime light pollution results from the inefficient use of lighting and wastes over $1 billion annually in the United States alone.

Because of light pollution, the vast majority of us rarely witness the majesty of the night sky. Of approximately 2,500 stars visible to the naked eye on a clear night, residents of major suburban areas can see only about 250 stars. From moderately sized urban areas, that number shrinks to approximately 50 stars. And from the center of a large city like New York or Chicago, we can see only about 15 stars on a clear night. The Milky Way, our own galactic neighborhood, is no longer visible to more than two-thirds of the United States population and half of the population of Europe.

Like air pollution, light pollution is most intense at its industrial, urban sources. But just as polluted air is blown around the globe, excessive nighttime lighting deflects beyond urban boundaries, resulting in a pernicious form of urban glow. Astronomer and light pollution expert Pierantonio Cinzano believes that 10 percent of the earth's population has compromised night vision as the result of such urban glow.

Recent studies indicate that 99 percent of the population of the Western world is exposed to varying degrees of light pollution. More than 95 percent of the population in the United States and the European Union lives in areas where the night sky is at least as bright as it is when there is a half moon. For those closer to the light sources, the sky remains nearly as bright as it is with a full moon. For 40 percent of the United States population, it never becomes dark enough at night for human eyes to adapt to night vision.

For most of us, then, even after we turn off the last lamp on our bed stand, night never fully arrives. Unless we take blackout measures, we are left with an eerie phosphorescent urban glow that seeps perniciously into our bedrooms. Considering the widespread use of nightlights and the proximity of illuminated clock radios, I believe that the majority of us suffer from a chronic darkness deficiency.

In one sense, the solution to light pollution is a simple one: turn down the lights. To reinstate night, we must deluminate our lives, our homes, our communities, the planet. In addition to having a positive impact on our health, delumination would help us restore our lost sense of rhythmicity and deliver significant economic benefits.

Although delumination is, in principle, a simple goal, I do not mean to suggest it is an easy one. Our communities are accustomed to and quite dependent on excessive LAN. Commercial and government operations also rely on a well-lit night world. Despite the fact that the benefits of delumination outweigh the costs on all fronts, we are left with our psychological resistance to experiencing darkness. But just as shadow work promises to reveal the diamonds in coal, so does delumination offer to reacquaint us with the forgotten magnificence of the night sky.

Geoff Chester, physicist and spokesman for the U.S. Naval Observatory, puts it simply: "The night sky is the world's largest national park with its stark beauty available to anyone who steps outside and looks up" (2001). As the result of light pollution and, I believe, the tantalizing distractions of modern entertainment options, far fewer people are witnessing the majesty of the night sky. Although we see things more clearly by day, we see significantly more depth by night—the very frame of our consciousness expands. The loss of this palpable experience of the heavens echoes the spiritual loss associated with the diminishment of night. Even with reduced visibility of stars, these are losses than we can begin to recoup by simply stepping outside.

"Night is a dead monotonous period under a roof," wrote Robert Louis Stevenson (1879, 26). The notion of thinking outside of the box is more than a metaphor. Like many others, I have observed a strong correlation between my immediate environment and the scope of my thinking. Many of the ideas presented in this book, for example, occurred to me during regular walks through the boundaries of darkness, at dusk and dawn. I wrote most of the original manuscript in the sanctuary of an old cathedral, whose spaciousness inspired more expansive thinking. As I was completing this closing chapter, I dreamed that I was back in that cathedral, which, surprisingly, had been restored to its original condition. I was struck by the fact that the sanctuary had a large gaping whole in the middle of its lofty ceiling. I could see the sky.

"Night is a dead monotonous period under a roof," continued Stevenson, "but in the open world it passes lightly, with its stars and dews and perfumes, and the hours are marked by changes in the face of Nature." For most of us, sunset is probably the most evident and accessible change in the face of night's Nature.

As an undergraduate at the University of Arizona in Tucson

in the late sixties, I participated in a community sunset-watching ritual. Two dozen or more students, hippies, hikers, and tourists would gather quietly on the craggy cliffs of Gates Pass, a desert mountain park just outside of the city that offered a vast, unobstructed western vista. We watched with awe as the face of Nature flushed pink in anticipation of the arrival of Nyx. A local FM radio station kindly coordinated a broadcast of "the sunset" in the form of the Beatles' song "Good Night," timing the event so that the song would end just as the sun sank beneath the horizon. Our silence was broken by oohs, aahs, and a hearty round of applause.

Such gatherings are common at various points around the globe where sunsets are particularly notable. Christopher Dewdney further examines this phenomenon in *Acquainted with the Night* (2004), an extraordinary exploration of the culture of night, suggesting a possible archetypal underpinning to our mesmerization by sunsets. Clearly, there is an almost sacred and religious dimension to such shared witnessing.

We need to redeem darkness, redefine our sense of night life. How can we create a greater forum for night in our lives? In addition to opening to night watching, we can add sunset watching, star gazing, moon watching, and intentionally developing a relationship with the night sky. What if telescopes became as ubiquitous as televisions?

Melatonin Replacement Therapy

Melatonin mediates our inner experience of darkness. It conveys a sense of night to our biology as well as to our consciousness. Modern lifestyles, however, significantly suppress our natural, endogenous melatonin levels. Just as we need to deluminate our homes, communities, and the world, I believe we also need to "deluminate" our biology and consciousness. Melatonin replacement therapy deserves serious consideration and further study from both a medical and a philosophical standpoint.

It is not difficult to understand why melatonin has been touted as a miracle substance. It is a complex and key player in our night biology, regulating circadian cycles, facilitating sleep, and promoting dreaming. Melatonin is also involved in the regulation of a wide range of hormones and neurotransmitters and functions as a potent antioxidant.

There is currently no consensus about what happens to our endogenous levels of melatonin as we age. Some studies suggest that melatonin levels decline with age, while others seem to contradict this. Without question, however, melatonin levels are adversely affected by numerous lifestyle factors. Just as light disrupts the still of night, a wide range of substances and medications tamper with our biological stillness by suppressing melatonin. Caffeine and alcohol both interfere with melatonin production. NSAIDs (nonsteroidal anti-inflammatory drugs), such as aspirin and ibuprofen, can decrease melatonin secretion in the body. Certain beta-blockers and diuretics can inhibit the nocturnal rise in melatonin. Benzodiazepine tranquilizers can also interfere with melatonin production. Additionally, electromagnetic fields, which occur in the vicinity of electrical devices such as bed stand clocks and electric blankets, can further suppress melatonin.

Other conditions permitting, the production and release of melatonin are stimulated by exposure to darkness and suppressed by light. Special sensors in our eyes keep the pineal gland informed about environmental light levels. Given that even relatively low levels of light can signal the brain to temporarily suppress melatonin production, it raises a critical question about what excessive and chronic overexposure to light at night does to one's melatonin.

Integrative medicine emphasizes the need for nutritional supplementation to compensate for the diminished nutrient value of our food as well as protect us against the excessive burden of toxic stressors associated with modern life. Likewise, we might consider compensating for our underexposure to darkness, our overexposure to excessive light at night, and the widespread suppression of melatonin associated with modern lifestyles by taking supplemental melatonin. Taking melatonin can help reverse the negative sleep side effects of medications such as beta-blockers, for example.

Replacing our suppressed melatonin may not be as simple as it sounds. Although melatonin replacement therapy can ultimately contribute to improved sleep and dreams, thinking of melatonin as a sleeping pill will probably lead to disappointment. Melatonin can help regulate our circadian rhythms and promote a kind of introverted relaxation, but no matter how much we take, it will not knock us out. Melatonin, like Nyx, brings dusk and night. And like night, melatonin does not insist that we sleep. It invites us to. Thinking of melatonin as the biological expression of Nyx also helps us recognize the spiritual and mythic dimensions of such supplementation.

I have two recommendations for those interested in melatonin replacement therapy. First, become informed. Although an in-depth discussion of melatonin is beyond the scope of this work, there is a large and growing body of accessible literature on the topic that is worthy of review. Second, find a knowledgeable health care professional to guide and support you in exploring important issues of safety, quality, and dosage.

What night offers the planet, melatonin provides for the person. It is darkness encoded in a molecule. By inviting dusk and darkness back into our bodies as well as our skies, we naturally invite the expression of our shadow issues. They no longer emerge opportunistically, sneaking in when our guard is down, but become an invited and intentional act of healing. The decision to deluminate is a decision to make peace with our shadows.

Integrating Consciousness

Except for Saturday afternoon naps, my father never slept. At least that was my hypothesis as a little boy. He was wide-awake when he tucked me in at night and then again when I caught sleepy glimpses of him silently praying over my bed at dawn. Because I never directly witnessed him retiring at night or arising in the morning, I surmised that he remained continuously awake. I was in awe of his stamina.

Waking is the gold standard for consciousness in our world.

In fact, for most of us, it is synonymous with consciousness. In contrast to waking, night consciousness and sleeping are parenthetical at best. We are waking-centric and have virtually no acceptable, coherent social framework for acknowledging the value and place of night consciousness, sleep, and dreams in our waking lives. People pictured in bed on television or film are rarely asleep. More often they are "sleeping together," but most often they are "lying awake together"—or alone.

Dreaming is the essential bridge between waking and sleeping—the resolution to the dialectic of night and day. Quick as it may be, we descend through a brief period of dreaming as we let go of waking and fall into sleep. At the other end, we normally awaken in the morning not directly from sleep but from dreaming. The dream also pulsates gently throughout our waking day, as the rest aspect of our basic rest and activity cycles. At night, sleep is our rest and dreaming is activity. By day, waking is activity and dreaming becomes our rest.

Dreaming is the refrain in the song of consciousness. As the story of Adam and Eve reminds us, life is but a dream. Dreaming occurs at the leading edge of each yin-yang wave. Where waking dissolves in sleep, we dream. And again where sleep transforms to waking, we dream. Dreaming is waking as seen through the sleeping body. And waking is a form of dreaming limited by the constraints of the world of matter. When we reinstate dreaming to its proper place in consciousness, we reconnect waking and sleeping and reestablish a sense of the sacred continuity of consciousness.

Our exploration of sleeping, dreaming, and waking has taught us that these states are not as discrete as we might have believed. Far from being a knockout, sleep emerges as the epitome of serenity—a way to get back home. We must reconceptualize sleep in terms of a continuum of tranquility that stretches from wakeful serenity to the unfathomable depths of slow-wave stillness.

A more honest definition of dreaming liberates it from night and sleep as well as from science and psychology. As we saw, we dream all the time. And dreaming is the essential antidote to lives choked by the exigencies of the mundane. A rapprochement with dreaming awakens us to the waking dream, enriching our lives with a palpable sense of spirituality, meaning, creativity, and deeper health.

Our expanded sense of night consciousness—of sleeping and dreaming—graciously reforms our sense of waking. We begin to realize that what we think of as waking is actually the product of both awareness and the object of our awareness. Nocturnal lucidity teaches us that the objects of awareness are not limited to the waking world and that aspects of night consciousness are a natural part of our days.

Ultimately, exploring the science and spirit of sleeping, dreaming, and waking is an inquiry into the essential nature of consciousness itself. We recognize that aspects of sleeping and dreaming are woven into our wakefulness, and that waking awareness waits patiently alongside of our sleep and dreams. We realize that all of these states of consciousness are present and available all the time.

They do not so much border one another, but overlap and integrate into a vibrant, rhythmic whole. At the deepest level, we are always experiencing all of these—simultaneously. Only through the segmentation of our awareness around night and night consciousness is the illusion of their separateness perpetuated. When we bring lucidity to night consciousness, we become aware of what it shares with day.

Like a braid of hair in which three separate strands weave together to form a whole, sleeping, dreaming, and waking are woven rhythmically into a single strand of consciousness. Although particular states may appear to be dominant at different times, each strand maintains a distinct identity, yet weaves together to form a larger whole.

The whole is greater than the sum of its parts. An integrated consciousness reaffirms the sacred union of the sun and moon, restoring balance and a sense of continuity or oneness to our lives. As we continue to bring greater lucidity to night and night consciousness, we observe an exquisite rhythmic order at play behind all things. We witness a grand and gracious sequential swirl of waking, sleeping, and dreaming throughout our days.

~

Our struggle for peace on Earth can ultimately be conceptualized as a struggle to come to terms with human consciousness, especially the dark and night consciousness aspect. In the end, an integrated consciousness is a more peaceful consciousness. I believe that we all know intuitively what my mother discovered in the Holocaust—that night itself is home to an innate peace. "Night, like peace," says Bruce Cockburn, "is a state of suspension" (1996).

Until recent years, with few exceptions, even military battles had to be suspended at night. Many indigenous cultures, particularly Native American tribes, abided by strict prohibitions against nighttime fighting. It was widely believed that dying at night made it difficult for a soul to find passage to the next world. With such prohibitions, there was a time for respite, for peace, even in the midst of war. Modern technology, however, has afforded us a new range of night vision options, high-tech ways of seeing in the dark. Today we have the option of engaging in battle 24/7.

One night while at her grandmother's home for dinner, my granddaughter, Claire, overheard a reference to war on an evening news broadcast. She grew visibly concerned and full of innocent curiosity about this most difficult subject. How does one discuss war with a four-year-old?

> "Bubby, they still have wars?" she asked.
> "Yes, Claire, it's very sad, but people still have wars."
> "Even now, Bubby, they have wars now?"
> "Yes, Claire, there are wars going on now."
> "People are fighting right *now*, Bubby?"
> "Yes, they are, sweetheart."
>
> Claire paused in confusion. "How could they? It's dark out."

Bibliography

Abrams, J. 1999. Shadow in America. *New Eyes Journal* 1 (1).

Barasch, M. 2000. *Healing dreams: Exploring the dreams that can transform your life.* New York: Riverhead.

Blask, D. E. 2003. Melatonin: An integrative chronobiotic anti-cancer therapy whose "time" has come? Presentation to the Program in Integrative Medicine, University of Arizona, March.

Blask, D. E., S. T. Wilson, and F. Zalatan. 1997. Physiological melatonin inhibition of human breast cancer cell growth in vitro: Evidence for a glutathione-mediated pathway. *Cancer Research* 57 (10).

Breggin, P. 2001. *The antidepressant fact book.* Cambridge, MA: Perseus.

Brower, K. J. 2001. Alcohol's effects on sleep in alcoholics. Bethesda, MD: National Institute on Alcohol Abuse and Alcoholism.

Brzezinski, A. 1997. Melatonin in humans. *New England Journal of Medicine* 336 (3).

Castaneda, C. 1993. *The art of dreaming.* New York: HarperCollins.

Center for Science in the Public Interest (CSPI). 1998. News release, Dec. 30. http://www.cspinet.org/new/sugar.htm.

Center for Science in the Public Interest (CSPI). 2005. http://www.cspinet.org.

Cherniske, S. 1998. *Caffeine blues: Wake up to the hidden dangers of America's #1 drug.* New York: Warner Books.

Chester, G. 2001. Starlight memories. *Washington Post,* Feb. 25.

Chodron, P. 2003. *Good medicine: How to turn pain into compassion with Tonglen meditation.* Louisville, CO: Sounds True.

Cockburn, B. 1996. *The charity of night.* Audio CD. Toronto: True North Records.

———. 1996. The mines of Mozambique. *The charity of night.* Audio CD. Toronto: True North Records.

Coren, S. 1996. *Sleep thieves: An eye-opening exploration into the science and mysteries of sleep.* New York: Free Press.

Dawson, D., and N. Encel. 1993. Melatonin and sleep in humans. *Journal of Pineal Research* 15: 1–12.

Dement, W. C., and C. Vaughan. 1999. *The promise of sleep: A pioneer in sleep medicine explains the vital connection between health, happiness, and a good night's sleep.* New York: Delacorte Press.

Dewdney, C. 2004. *Acquainted with the night: Excursions through the world after dark.* Toronto: HarperCollins.

Domhoff, G. W. 2003. *The scientific study of dreams.* Washington, DC: American Psychological Association.

Edison, T. A., and D. D. Runes, eds. 1948. *The diary and sundry observations of Thomas Alva Edison.* New York: Philosophical Library.

Ekirch, A. R. 2005. *At day's close: Night in times past.* New York: W. W. Norton.

Estes, C. P. 1992. *Women who run with the wolves.* New York: Ballantine.

Evans, E. 1926. *A psychological study of cancer.* New York: Dodd, Mead.

Ford, D. 1998. *The dark side of the light chasers: Reclaiming your power, creativity, brilliance, and dreams.* New York: Riverhead.

Forman, R. K. 1999. *Mysticism, mind, consciousness.* Ithaca: State University of New York Press.

Foster, H. D. 2000. Why schizophrenics who smoke have a lower incidence of lung cancer: Implications for the treatment of both disorders. *Journal of Orthomolecular Medicine* 15 (3).

Frankiel, T., and J. Greenfield. 2000. *Entering the temple of dreams.* Woodstock, VT: Jewish Lights Publishing.

Fredholm, B., K. Bättig, J. Holmén, A. Nehlig, and E. Zvartau. 1999. Actions of caffeine in the brain with special reference to factors that contribute to its widespread use. *Pharmacological Reviews* 51 (1) (March): 83–133.

Gackenbach, J. 1988. From sleep consciousness to pure consciousness. Presidential address to the annual meeting of the Association for the Study of Dreams. London. www.sawka.com/spiritwatch/from.htm.

Gleick, J. 1999. *Faster: The acceleration of just about everything.* New York: Pantheon.

Greenbaum, A. 1993. *The sweetest hour: Tikkun chatzot.* Jerusalem/New York: Breslov Research Institute.

Harnack, L., J. Stang, and M. Story. 1999. Soft drink consumption among U.S. children and adolescents: Nutritional consequences. *Journal of the American Dietetic Association* 99 (4): 436–41.

Hill, S. M., and D. E. Blask. 1988. Effects of the pineal hormone melatonin on the proliferation and morphological characteristics of human breast cancer cells (MCF-7) in culture. *Cancer Research* 48 (21).

Hillman, J. 1979. *The dream and the underworld.* New York: Harper and Row.

Holy Bible, King James Version. 1972. Nashville: Thomas Nelson Publishers.

Honoré, C. 2004. *In praise of slowness.* New York: HarperCollins.

Hrushesky, W., D. Blask, P. Lissoni. 2003. Melatonin, chronobiology, and cancer. NCI Office of Cancer Complementary and Alternative Medicine, Invited Speaker Series.

International Dark-Sky Association. Tucson. www.darksky.org.

Jacobs, G. D. 1998. *Say goodnight to insomnia.* New York: Henry Holt.

Jacobson, M. F. 1998. Liquid candy: How soft drinks are harming Americans' health. Washington, DC: Center for Science in the Public Interest.

Kalff, D. 1980. *Sandplay.* Boston: Sigo Press.

Kripke, D. F. 1997–2002. *The dark side of sleeping pills.* San Diego. www.thedarksideofsleepingpills.com.

———. 2002. *Brighten your life.* San Diego. www.brightenyourlife.info.

Kryger, M. H., T. Roth, and W. C. Dement. 2000. *Principles and practices of sleep medicine*. Philadelphia: W. B. Saunders.

Lambert G. W., C. Reid, D. M. Kaye, G. L. Jennings, and M. D. Esler. 2002. Effect of sunlight and season on serotonin turnover in the brain. *Lancet* 360: 1840–42.

Levine, S. 1989. *A gradual awakening*. New York: Anchor.

Lynch, E. M. 2004. Melatonin and cancer treatment. *Life Extension Magazine*. Hollywood, FL: Life Extension Foundation.

Maas, James. 1998. *Power sleep*. New York: Villard.

Malhotra, S., G. Sawhney, and P. Pandhi. 2004. The therapeutic potential of melatonin: A review of the science. *Medscape General Medicine* 6 (2).

Mindell, A. 1993. *The shaman's body*. San Francisco: Harper.

———. 2000. *Dreaming while awake*. Charlottesville, VA: Hampton Roads.

Moldofsky, H. 1995. Sleep, neuroimmune and neuroendocrine functions in fibromyalgia and chronic fatigue syndrome. *Advances in Neuroimmunology* 5 (1).

Moore, T. 1992. *Care of the soul: A guide for cultivating depth and sacredness in everyday life*. New York: HarperCollins.

Muller, W. 1999. *Sabbath: Restoring the scared rhythm of rest*. New York: Bantam.

National Coffee Association of USA. 2000. NCA Coffee Drinking Trends Survey, 2000. New York.

National Commission on Sleep Disorders Research. 2005. http://www.stanford.edu/~dement/overview-ncsdr.html.

National Highway Traffic Safety Administration. 2005. http://www.nhtsa.dot.gov/.

National Sleep Foundation. 1994–2005. Sleep in America Poll. www.sleepfoundation.org.

Nhat Hanh, T. 2001. *Thich Nhat Hanh: Essential writings*. Maryknoll, NY: Orbis Books.

Olgive, R. D., and J. R. Harsh. 1994. *Sleep onset: Normal and abnormal processes*. Washington, DC: American Psychological Association.

Ott, J. 2000. *Health and light: The effects of natural and artificial light on man and other living things.* Boston: Ariel Press.

Pendergrast, M. 2000. *Uncommon grounds: The history of coffee and how it transformed our world.* New York: Basic Books.

Prather, H. 2000. *The little book of letting go.* Berkeley, CA: Conari Press.

————. 2005. *Morning notes: 365 meditations to wake you up.* Boston: Conari Press.

Prather, H., and G. Prather. 1991. *Parables from other planets.* New York: Bantam.

Pressman, M. R., and W. C. Orr, eds. 1997. *Understanding sleep: The evaluation and treatment of sleep disorders.* Washington, DC: American Psychological Association.

Reiter, R., and J. Robinson. 1995. *Melatonin: Your body's natural wonder drug.* New York: Bantam.

Rock, A. 2004. *The mind at night: The new science of how and why we dream.* New York: Basic Books.

Rossi, E. L., and D. Nimmons 1991. *The 20-minute break.* Los Angeles: Tarcher.

Rumi, J. 1981. *Night and sleep.* Trans. R. Bly. Somerville, MA: Yellow Moon Press.

Rychlak, J. F. 2003. *The human image in postmodern America.* Washington, DC: American Psychological Association.

Sahelian, R. 1995. *Melatonin: Nature's sleeping pill.* Marina Del Rey, CA: Be Happier Press.

Skully, N. 2003. *Alchemical healing: A guide to spiritual, physical, and transformational medicine.* Rochester, VT: Bear and Company.

Solms, M., and O. Turnbull. 2003. *Comparison of dreaming to schizophrenic delusion in brain and the inner world: An introduction to the neuroscience of subjective experience.* New York: Other Press.

Staudenmaier, J. M. 1996. Denying the holy dark: The enlightenment ideal and the European mystical tradition. In *Progress: Fact or illusion?* ed. Leo Marx and Bruce Mazlish. Ann Arbor: University of Michigan Press.

Steiner, R., and M. Lipson, eds. 2003. *Sleep and dreams: A bridge to the spirit.* Great Barrington, MA: Steiner Books.

Stevenson, R. L. 1879. *Travels with a donkey in the Cevennes.* Classic Literature Library. www.classic-literature.co.uk.

Szuba, M. P., ed. 2001. *Depression and anxiety: The psychobiology of sleep and major depression.* New York: Wiley-Liss.

Terman, M. 1997. Light on sleep. In *Scientific foundations of sleep therapies,* ed. W. J. Schwartz. Basel: Karger.

Terman, M., and D. S. Schlager. 1990. Twilight therapeutics, winter depression, melatonin, and sleep. In *Sleep and biological rhythms,* ed. J. Montplaisir and R. Godbout. New York: Oxford University Press.

Terman, M., D. Schlager, S. Fairhurst, and B. Perlman. 1989. Dawn and dusk simulation as a therapeutic intervention. *Biological Psychiatry* 25: 966–70.

Thayer, R. E. 2001. *Calm energy: How people regulate mood with food and exercise.* New York: Oxford University Press.

Thoreau, H. D. 1854. *Walden; or, Life in the woods.* theliteraturepage .com.

Varela, F. J. 1997. *Sleeping, dreaming, and dying: An exploration of consciousness with the Dalai Lama.* Boston: Wisdom Publications.

Vgontzas, A. N., E. Zoumakis, E. O. Bixler, H.-M. Lin, H. Follett, A. Kales, and G. P. Chrousos. 2004. Adverse effects of modest sleep restriction on sleepiness, performance, and inflammatory cytokines. *Journal of Clinical Endocrinology and Metabolism* 89 (5).

Wangyal, T. 1998. *The Tibetan yogas of dream and sleep.* Ithaca, NY: Snow Lion Publications.

Watkins, M. 1976. *The waking dream.* Dallas: Spring Publications.

Wehr, T. A. 1999. The impact of changes in nightlength (scotoperiod) on human sleep. In *Neurobiology of sleep and circadian rhythms,* ed. F. W. Turek and P. C. Zee, 263–85. New York: Marcel Dekker.

Weil, A. 1980. *The marriage of the sun and moon: A quest for unity in consciousness.* Boston: Houghton Mifflin.

———. 1995. *Spontaneous healing.* New York: Knopf.

Wiley, T. S., and B. Formby. 2000. *Lights out: Sleep, sugar, and survival.* New York: Pocket Books.

Winterson, J. 1998. *The world and other places.* New York: Vintage Books.

Yun, A. J., K. A. Bazar, A. Gerber, P. Y. Lee, and S. M. Daniel. 2005. The dynamic range of biologic functions and variation of many environmental cues may be declining in the modern age: Implications for diseases and therapeutics. *Medical Hypotheses* 65 (1): 173–78. Epub Jan. 5.

Zehme, Bill. 1994. Inside the mind of Dave. *Esquire,* December.

Zhdanova, I. V., H. J. Lynch, and R. J. Wurtman. 1997. Melatonin: A sleep promoting hormone. *Sleep* 20 (10).

Zweig, C., and J. Abrams, eds. 1991. *Meeting the shadow.* Los Angeles: Tarcher.

Index

To order additional copies of *Healing Night*

Web: www.itascabooks.com

Phone: 1-800-901-3480

Fax: Copy and fill out the form below with credit card information. Fax to 763-398-0198.

Mail: Copy and fill out the form below. Mail with check or credit card information to:

Syren Book Company
5120 Cedar Lake Road
Minneapolis, MN 55416

Order Form

Copies	Title / Author	Price	Totals
	Healing Night / **Rubin R. Naiman, Ph.D.**	$14.95	$
	Subtotal		$
	7% sales tax (MN only)		$
	Shipping and handling, first copy		$ 4.00
	Shipping and handling, ___ add'l copies @$1.00 ea.		$
	TOTAL TO REMIT		$

Payment Information:

__ Check Enclosed __ Visa/MasterCard		
Card number:	Expiration date:	
Name on card:		
Billing address:		
City:	State:	Zip:
Signature:	Date:	

Shipping Information:

__ Same as billing address __ Other (enter below)		
Name:		
Address:		
City:	State:	Zip: